Lucky One

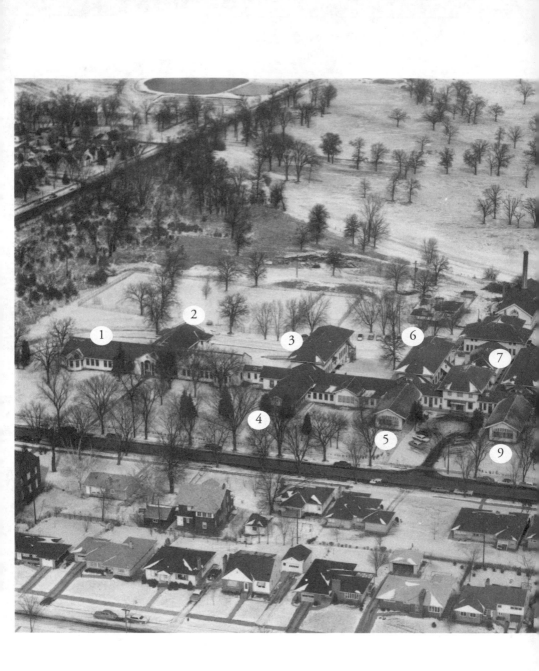

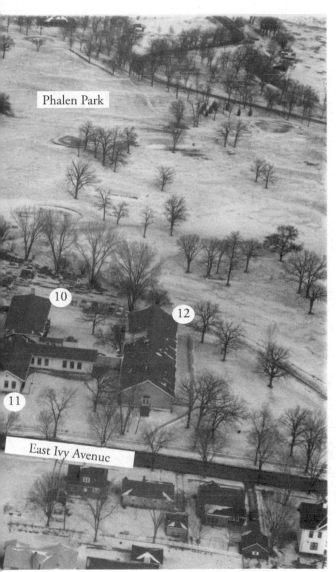

Phalen Park

East Ivy Avenue

Gillette State Hospital for
Crippled Children in 1959:

1 classrooms

2 auditorium

3 Wards 2 and 3
(little children)

4 Ward 1
(older boys, bed)

5 Ward 5
(young boys, up and bed)

6 Ward 6
(older boys, up)

7 kitchen

8 Ward 8
(older girls, up)

9 Ward 7
(young girls, up and bed)

10 surgery

11 Ward 9
(older girls, bed)

12 new admitting unit
(main level);
outpatient unit and
playroom (lower level)

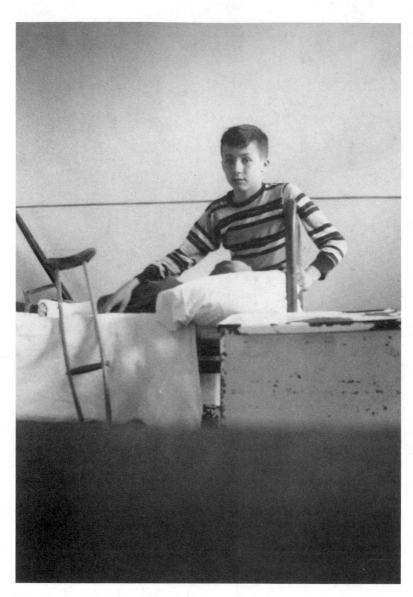

In bed in 1952–53 following one of the operations on my right foot

Lucky One

Making It Past Polio and Despair

Richard Maus

luckyonebook.com

ANTERIOR PUBLISHING

Northfield, Minnesota

Published by: luckyonebook.com
an imprint of Anterior Publishing
204 West 7th Street, Box 8
Northfield, MN 55057
507-645-4633
author@luckyonebook.com

Author photo: John Danicic, Jr.
Cover photo: Benjamin Hillis
Editor: Nancy Ashmore, Ashmore Ink
Book design: Dorie McClelland, Spring Book Design
Cover design: Amy Kirkpatrick
Photo credits:
    Aerial photo inside cover, *St. Paul Dispatch & Pioneer Press,*
        Minnesota Historical Society
    Ward 6 photo, page 32, A.F. Raymond, Minnesoa Historical Society
    Entry record, page 5, Minnesota Historical Society

Printed in the United States of America
11 10 09 08 07 06   2 3 4 5 6 7 8
First Edition

ISBN: 0-9776205-0-6

To Donna, Paul, and Steve

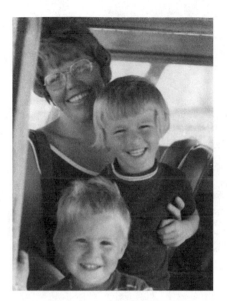

In our airplane in 1973

Acknowledgments

I am grateful to the following for their encouragement and their suggestions, small and large. They have made this a better book. Any mistakes that remain are mine.

John Andrisen, Deane Barbour, Faith Bergemann, Phyllis Borchert, Nora De Master, Peter Doughty, Audrey Ebert, Amy Farrar, James Froom, Mary Gardner, Liz Hankins, Barb Havel, Dave Havel, Linda Hunter, Eileen Keller, Laurie LaMoore, Solvig Land, Elizabeth Larson, Hope Lavine, Walt Lee, Constance Lepro, Donna Maus, Louise Maus, Paul Maus, Phil Maus, Ruth Maus Rothschilds, Steve Maus, Jane McWilliams, Lydia Quanbeck Moe, Kathy Paige, Marian Phelps, Jim Reiley, Tom Rogalski, Connie Sansome, Jean Seely, Hollida Wakefield Underwager, and Joy Wolf.

Acceptance is hard.
To accept my pain means holding it in
my arms, like a package handed to me,
my proper burden to be carried.
The package may be heavy as lead,
or burning hot,
or stuck through with razors,
but I must concede that it is my
package, simply because it has arrived
in my life.
It is not a mistake.
It has not been sent by accident
to the wrong person.
I may not welcome it, but accepting it
means I carry it without protest
for as long as necessary—
and then I lay it down.

JEANNE DuPRAU
The Earth House (1990)

Prologue

I have wanted to tell this story all my life.

This memoir is my version of my young life, shaped by the fact that I contracted polio when I was a baby.

I've tried to be factual about what it was like to grow up in the 1940s, 50s, and 60s. I've included details of dairy farming, orthopedic surgery, educational miscalculations, combining wheat, highway construction, flying, and teaching, but I haven't presented the whole story. I have omitted many significant but common nonessential life events in the interest of better storytelling. To preserve the privacy of a few individuals, I have altered some names.

Although the chapters contain excerpts from my medical records from Gillette State Hospital for Crippled Children and the end of the book includes a fuller accounting of the care I received there, you can read *Lucky One* with or without the clinical information.

Keep in mind as you read this story that the medical treatment I received and the events I describe took place a half century ago. Times have changed since then and largely for the better.

There are also aspects of this story that are timeless. Writing this book has taught me much about things that are worth affirming and about things that haven't changed but should. I hope it will do the same for you.

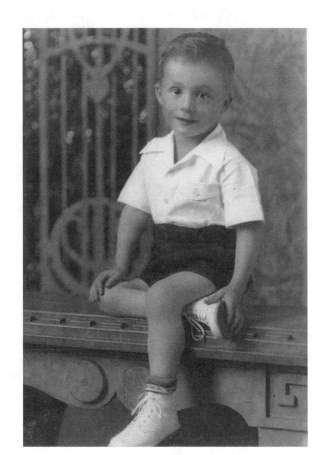

My first formal portrait, age four

*W*hen the doctor arrived at our old farmhouse in central Minnesota at mid-afternoon on August 21, 1939, I was well into the second day of a flu-like illness. Mother and Dad had sent for him, concerned about my high fever and constant crying. They had tried to soothe me, but when they touched anywhere on my 4-month-old body, I just screamed louder.

"Looks like he has the summer complaint," the doctor said. "All you can do is try to control the fever with cool, wet towel packs."

I didn't sleep much that day or the next. Neither did my parents, Benno and Lorrayne Maus. They were frantic. I couldn't be of any help, either. All I knew was that it hurt.

By the fourth day, there were signs of improvement. I slept some and was not as sensitive to touch. In a few more days, I ate and slept normally. The crisis had passed.

Life returned to normal. The grain harvest was finished and the threshing crew of neighbors had disbanded. Mother went back to running the household and the annual task of canning fruits and vegetables. Dad tended to outdoor chores, taking care of the cows, pigs, and horses. The chickens took care of themselves, scratching for dropped oats around the new straw pile and where the threshing machine had stood. It was a good time to replace broken windows in the barn and fix fences around the fields and pastures.

A month after my illness I was bouncing in a canvas Johnny-jump-up hanging in the doorway between the kitchen and the dining room. My sister Ruth Ann, a year older than I, was in a playpen off to the side. While we played, Mother hurried about the kitchen baking bread and preparing noon lunch. Cooler weather was coming and the world looked better. She had her children nearby. They were healthy.

A casual glance my way turned into several. I seemed to be doing more work with one of my legs than the other. Was the right one lazy or maybe tired? Did I take turns using one leg then the other?

Dad came in from watering and unharnessing the horses, Tom and Jerry. "Watch his legs," Mother said. "Do you notice anything?"

"He might be using the left leg a little more," Dad finally observed.

Everything else seemed fine. I was passing a toy back and forth with my hands. My temperature and appetite were normal. I was alertly watching everything going on around me in the kitchen.

They had never studied a child's legs that closely before. "Maybe they sometimes use one more than another," Dad suggested. "Like a lefty favoring a left hand?"

During the week that followed, they noticed that my right foot seemed to hang more and the left foot pushed more. It was becoming clear that something was affecting the right leg.

"I think we should take him to Albany," Dad declared.

Mother quickly agreed. The doctor who had seen me a month earlier might not be as helpful as Aloys Mahowald, Dad's brother-in-law, a physician with a practice in Albany, 40 miles north of our farm in Watkins.

It didn't take Dr. Mahowald long to figure out what was happening. He only had to examine my leg and hear about the illness I'd had in August.

"He has polio," he announced.

He tried to be reassuring, but the diagnosis came like a thunderbolt. Everyone in the country was afraid of polio. Everybody knew someone crippled with it. It had permanently paralyzed President Roosevelt's legs. It put people in iron lungs. It killed children. Nobody knew, however, how the poliovirus was transmitted or how long you were contagious if you got it.

"What do we do now?" asked Dad, glancing at my mother.

"Some muscles in the baby's right leg are not working," said the doctor. "Because of the poliovirus, the muscles that pull up the front of the foot are not getting activating nerve signals, but the muscles connected to the heel cord are. That means the foot will be pulled down in front as the leg grows."

"He will need medical attention or the problem will get worse," he continued. "A bad leg problem can result in a back problem."

Dad squirmed. He did not have much money. Our small 80-acre farm at the northeast edge of Watkins, a rural town west of Minneapolis, Minnesota, could barely support our family and the horses it took to operate it. He was renting the place from his sister, Hedwig. She and her husband, Henry Johnson, had bought the farm from their father, John A. Maus, when he retired from teaching, farming, and raising a family of 12 children and moved to Spring Hill.

"Let me check, but I think we can get Richard into Gillette Hospital," Dr. Mahowald continued. "Gillette has the best doctors for this condition. It won't cost you anything, but you will have to agree to let them be in charge of his treatment."

Gillette State Hospital for Crippled Children was funded by the Minnesota State Legislature. It took its name from the man who had served as its first surgeon-in-chief, Dr. Arthur Gillette. Before that it was known as the Minnesota State Hospital for Indigent, Crippled and Deformed Children.

Care was free at Gillette Hospital. Experienced orthopedic surgeons essentially donated the time they spent working with patients who had problems with their bones, joints, or muscles. It was located 80 miles from Watkins, near Lake Phalen in St. Paul.

Dad nodded tersely. He was relieved that they would be able to get good help for me but frightened by all the unknowns that lay ahead. The drive home was a quiet and solemn one.

A letter soon arrived from Gillette. It stated that I had been accepted for treatment and should come to the hospital to be admitted. On Thursday, November 2, 1939, at the age of six months, I would become a ward of the state for my medical treatment.

Mother and I headed for Gillette early that morning in November. My father stayed behind to help take care of Ruth Ann and tend to the farm animals.

The trip took two hours, one on Highway 55, the 60 miles of graveled, dusty road between Watkins to Robbinsdale, and another of stop-and-go city driving. It must have seemed even longer to Mother. She was preparing to leave her baby in the care of a hospital that she had never seen and with people that she knew very little about.

What was the treatment for polio? How long would I have to be there? My mother didn't know. She only knew that she wouldn't be there with me. Even if hospital practice permitted parents to stay with their children while they were in the hospital, and it didn't, she had responsibilities on the farm and a toddler to take care of.

306

STATE OF MINNESOTA
GILLETTE HOSPITAL FOR CRIPPLED CHILDREN
Phalen Park, St. Paul, Minnesota

Name *Richard Maus* No. *5485*

1st ad. Admitted *11-2- 19 39* *9* Hour *A.* M

Age *6 months* Sex *M.* Nationality *Am.* Grade in School *No school*

Date of Birth *4.24.39* Birth Place *Watkins, Minn*

Birth Place of Parents Father *Albany, Minn* Mother *Watkins, Minn*

Religion *Catholic*

Residence *Watkins, Minn* County *Meeker*

Name and P. O. address of Father, Mother, or nearest friend or relative
Benno Maus
Lorrayne Geislinger Maus

Brought to Hospital by *mother*

From *home*

Cause of Admission *Residual Poliomyelitis, right foot (Onset Aug 20, 1939)*

Services of Doctor *Chatterton + von der Weyer*

Treatment, Operation, Date, etc. *Blood Wasserman + Mantzer test negative Neurological examination by Dr. Kamman 1-28-39 Splint Physiotherapy.*

Appliances *Short leg brace, right, attached to shoe.*

Result *Improved*

Discharged, Med — *8-10- 19 40* Time in Hospital *314*

Have Permission to operate *√*

Remarks

First admissions entry, 1939, Gillette State Hospital for Crippled Children

5

Mother wasn't at the hospital very long. She answered the doctor's questions as he examined me. She held me in her lap as he explained that in the months to come they would put splints on my right leg, replacing them as I grew. The half casts made of plaster would push up the front of my foot to counter the tug of the heel cord. She hoped it wouldn't be as painful as it sounded. I would be kept in isolation to make sure I didn't infect other patients. She was welcome to see me during visiting hours, he told her, but now it was time for the nurse to take me to the ward.

After a goodbye that was much too quick, Mother returned to the car. Months! We were going to be apart for months! She thought about all the "firsts" she was going to miss. The first time I stood by myself. Playing patty-cake and waving bye-bye. Saying "mama" and "dada." My first teeth. Maybe even taking my first steps. Putting the car in gear, she began the long, tearful journey home.

MEDICAL HISTORY 11-2-1939
Family history negative for orthopedic abnormalities, tuberculosis, cancer, and diabetes. No operations and no injuries. Diagnosis on admission – Residual Poliomyelitis, right foot (Onset August 20, 1939)

The patient is a well developed, well nourished child, six months of age. At present in no acute distress.

In the right leg there is some muscular atrophy due to Poliomyelitis. Patient has, however, still a little motion in the leg.

Admitted to Ward 2 at 1:30 P.M. Isolated in cubicle. Given routine admission care. Splint applied to right foot as ordered. No teeth.

Meanwhile, I was taken to Ward 2, isolation, where white-gowned nurses with protective masks on their faces introduced me to my new home. The stark cubicle was large enough to hold a crib and to allow the doctor to examine me and the nurses to diaper, dress, and feed me. A window on one side enabled them to check on me throughout the day. It was also the only way visitors could see me.

Mother and Dad arranged to come and visit me every two weeks to check on my medical status. By early December, when they made their second visit, they could not get my attention from the other side of the glass. I did not know them anymore.

Figuring that it made no sense to make a four-hour round trip and inconvenience the friends who were tending to farm chores in their stead in order to visit someone who would not even look up at them, they reluctantly discontinued their visits. I was 7 months old.

I spent six months in Ward 2 learning the routines and getting to know the staff. I was vaccinated for whooping cough and got a fever. They put a new long leg plaster on my right leg, then a metal night brace, then a posterior plaster splint. I was "active and happy," according the medical records, and by mid-January I weighed 18 pounds.

At the end of April, the month I turned one, I was transferred to Ward 3. I was active, the nurses said. By mid-July I was standing up in my crib and I had two teeth. The same month they made a new splint to be used at night and then a long leg brace of lightweight steel that could be attached to a shoe. In August the records noted that I had been "seen walking."

5-5-1940
Weight 19 pounds, 11 ounces. Gaining weight. Eats well.
Happy. Plays by himself.

6-16-1940

Appetite is very good. Tries to stand up in bed.

7-7-1940

Is very active. Stands up in his crib. Has two teeth.

8-29-1940

Seen walking. Is walking fairly well.

A month later, the hospital decided I was ready to be sent home. At 4:35 P.M. on Tuesday, September 10, 1940, I was "discharged to mother." Before she carried me to the car through the damp of a cool fall day, they taught her my exercises and showed her how the brace and splint fit on my leg. I had been at Gillette for 314 days. I was not quite 1½ years old. I returned to a home that I was much too young to have any memory of and to a family of strangers, including a sister I had never met, Helen, born a month earlier.

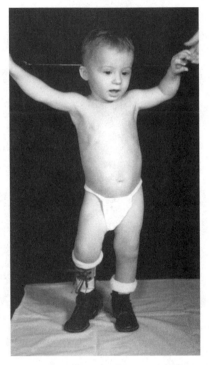

Getting ready to go home with first brace, after 11 months at Gillette

The first week was a tough one. Mother and Dad were happy to have me home again, but whenever they approached me, to pick me up, help me, or dress me, I screamed in terror. I not only did not know them, I feared them.

On Sunday after Mother left the house for church, the only one in town, Dad had an idea. He went to the bedroom closet and found a white shirt and a washed-out, nearly white pair of slacks. He put these on and walked out to the kitchen. When he approached me, I eagerly put out my arms. I wanted Dad to pick me up.

He was still standing in the kitchen, his arms wrapped tenderly around me, my arm around his neck, when Mother came home.

"What did you do?" she exclaimed. He didn't answer. He didn't have to. The solution was obvious and reassuring in a way. It indicated that I had been treated well at the hospital. That I had felt safe there.

Mother and Dad decided to dress like doctors and nurses until I learned to accept them again. It took a few days.

They had to make other adjustments as well. Mother often told how the nurse had showed her how to teach me to get out of my crib. To her surprise, before she could do so I got out on my own.

I continued to grow—and to outgrow the devices that had been designed to counter the constant tug of the heel cord on my right foot. They made me a new splint in December and a new brace in March 1941, checking regularly to see that they fit and worked as intended.

4-17-1941

The foot is in good position. There is practically no anterior tibial function. To have plaster model made for new castex night splint, right foot. To have new shoes. ... To report in 6 months.

8-28-1941

The right heel is being drawn up by a short heel cord and he has a semi-rocker type of foot. Mother is to apply hot packs to right lower leg. Discontinue the brace, but get him a new metal night splint. To report in three months.

11-19-1942

The right foot cannot be brought up to within 10° or 15° of the
right angle, and the foot is pronated. Put in a light spring steel
in the sole of the right shoe and build up the inner edge of the
heel and sole 1/8 inch, light leather arch in shoe. Continue
with the check strap on the right shoe. To report in February
or March 1943.

After two years, it became obvious that this course of treatment was
not working. The foot did not make a right angle with the lower leg. At
age four, I could walk, run and climb, but on my right foot only the toes
touched the ground.

The doctors decided that the heel cord should be lengthened surgically. I was readmitted to Gillette on April 20, 1944. Four days later, on
my fifth birthday, I had my first operation. This time I would be in the
hospital for a total of 85 days.

4-24-1944

OPERATION: Open lengthening of tendo Achilles, right. Under
general anesthesia, an incision approximately 2 inches long
was made along the medial side of the right tendo Achilles, and,
by dull dissection, the tendon was dissected out of the subcutaneous fat. Anterior-posterior Z plasty was done. The tendon
was lengthened enough to bring the foot to just beyond a right
angle, and re-sutured with interrupted sutures of chromic
catgut. The fascia was closed with plain catgut, and the skin
with black silk interrupted sutures. Sterile dressings were
applied, followed by plaster of Paris cast extending from the
mid thigh to include the toes.

Returned to Ward at 10:50 A.M. in good condition. Right leg elevated. Circulation, sensation, and motion in toes good. Given Codeine grains 1/2 at 2:30 P.M. Slept well during the night. No complaints.

My earliest memory of Gillette dates from this period. Unlike later hospitalizations, however, my recollection is not of the operation or the hardships of recovering from it. What I remember is being in the auditorium, in a bed, watching cartoons on a big movie screen. The place was full of kids in beds.

I also remember being terrified every night by giants thumping around outside the hospital. Sometimes they seemed to be looking for me. Other times a single giant might get up and thump away toward the horizon. I seldom fell asleep while I could hear them.

Thump. Thump. Thump. Thump. They got louder, nearer, and faster. Under the covers I went. "It's dark," I whispered to myself. "Lie still. Don't move. Wait. If you remain motionless long enough, they'll go away. They always do."

My heart thumped so loudly I was sure it could be heard. I was afraid my breathing was audible, too. I shook with a fear that was barely under control.

The night nurse working at her desk near a lamp appeared unbothered by the giants, however, and inside the ward, all was quiet.

Finally it sounded like only one giant was left, and it seemed to be leaving. I could barely hear it. Yes, it was gone.

I came out from under the sheets. Everything seemed safe. They hadn't gotten me this time, but they'd come back. They always did.

Still, staring at the dimly lit ceiling I felt lucky to have survived the encounter. Gradually I relaxed and fell to sleep.

The thumping-giant nightmares often lasted more than an hour.

7-13-1944
Discharged, improved; to report in October.
Discharged to his aunt at 2 P.M. ... Wearing shoes with check
strap on (right) shoe.

Finally I was ready to go home again. Aunt Hedwig, who lived in
Minneapolis, came to pick me up and take me to the farm. I still today
remember getting out of her car to my welcome home. Things weren't as
awkward as when I was a toddler probably, but I had spent nearly three
months in the hospital. Things felt different, strange, and so did I.

That night Mother, Dad, Ruth (age six), Helen (almost four) and I
sat in the kitchen, relaxing and waiting for bedtime. Philip, who was
one, was in bed already. Ruth and Helen were taking turns sitting on
the foot of Dad's crossed leg, bouncing up and down playing horsy.
They seemed to be having lots of fun. I looked silently on. Dad coaxed
me to try it, too, but I did not want to. I just wanted to watch. I didn't
know why.

Finally it was time for bed. Mother offered each of us a treat, a piece
of banana, along with a nighttime kiss. My sisters quickly accepted. I
didn't. I did not want to kiss her goodnight. She sent me to bed without
the treat. I was sad and angry about that for a long time.

I endured a few more upsets before life got back to normal. I also
experienced a revelation. It occurred in the farmyard.

The Soo Line passed through Watkins on its way from Minneapolis
to Winnipeg. The tracks went straight past our farm. Four passenger
trains and many long freights rumbled by every day. You could hear the
steam engines long before you saw them. The sound had a surprising

effect on me after I returned from the hospital. It made my body shake. My blood turned cold and seemed to flow down my legs. Before the train came into view, I was hiding behind the nearest tree or building.

I was watching a locomotive chug by one day when I suddenly recognized what the sounds reminded me of. They were the thumps of my nighttime "giants." The Lake Phalen region of St. Paul was filled with railroad tracks and my 5-year-old's mind had interpreted the deep choo, choo, choo, choo of steamers moving freight as the footsteps of lumbering monsters. Each thump was a giant foot, hitting the ground, taking another step out there in the dark.

It took a few weeks but eventually I no longer felt the need to hide when a train went by. Later I became quite fascinated with them.

8-30-44
Right shoe built up and mailed.

10-26-44
The patient still has slight equinus of the right foot, pes planus, and the arch of the shoe should be reinforced with a short steel ... Mother was instructed to continue manipulating the foot every day, and when he gets new shoes to send in the right one to be altered. Patient to report in the spring.

11-8-44
Shoe built up and mailed.

6-7-45
Shoe built up and mailed to patient.

7-11-45
Shoe built up and mailed.

Finally, it was time to get ready for school. Ruth was in the second grade. I would be in first. Helen, waiting impatiently, wouldn't start until the following year.

Mother made all our clothes, everything except the underwear and socks, using a foot pedal-powered sewing machine. I helped pick up supplies like paper and crayons.

A few days before classes began, Mother and I went to school. While she and my teacher visited, I poked my fingers into the raised sandbox in the classroom.

I couldn't tell what they were talking about, but I sensed it was about me. About whether I was ready to start the next chapter of my life. I thought I was.

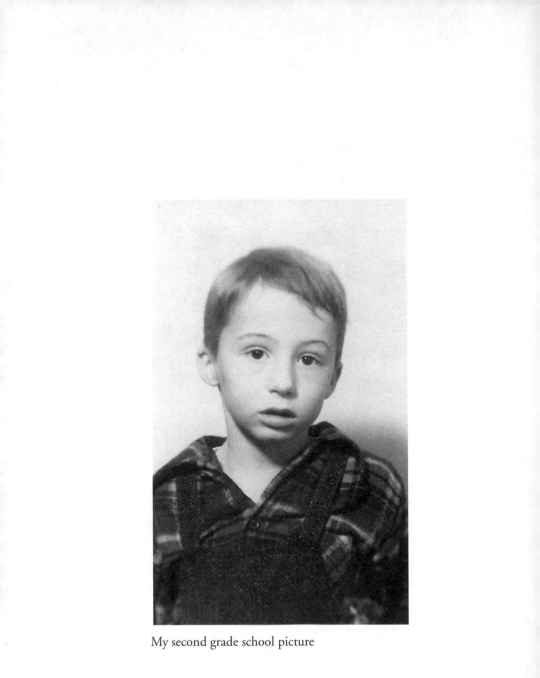

My second grade school picture

*t*hat first year of school produced indelible memories—some good and some bad.

One of the best took place early in the school year. It was Saturday morning, and my mother was in the kitchen with Mary Ann Bauer, the hired girl. Almost 18, she came to the house every day to help Mother with household work and childcare.

I don't know where my sisters and baby brother were, but I was in the entry room, playing on the sun-warmed floor. During my recent hospital stay, I'd learned how to entertain myself.

As Mother and Mary Ann ironed and folded the baskets of laundry that had been dried on the clothesline the day before, I daydreamed and marked the progress of the sun across the floor. Whenever I noticed that the warm, bright spot defined by the window frame had moved, I nudged my toy truck to mark its new edge.

This continued quietly for hours. Did Mother and Mary Ann even remember I was there? If not, it must have been a big surprise when suddenly I burst into song.

"Life is but a dream," I warbled.

There was a pause, and then the two of them went wild with laughter. I don't remember ever hearing my mother laugh so long and so hard.

"What did you say?" asked Mother. To my delight, she was still laughing.

"Life is but a dream," I sang again.

"Where did you get that?" she said, still a little breathless.

"In school yesterday we were singing 'Row Row Row Your Boat.' Each row of desks would start singing at a different place. One row started, then the next until all the rows were singing the same song but at different places. It was fun. I was singing the song to myself and at the end I just sang it out loud. I wish we would sing that every day."

Life in rural Minnesota certainly had its dream-like qualities in 1945, especially if you were too young to have daily chores. Watkins had a church, a parochial school, a post office, a bank, a creamery, a cheese plant, a movie theater, three grocery stores, five bars, and assorted other businesses. Our farm was on the northeast edge of town, just four or five blocks from school. When class let out every day, we'd walk slowly home, in small, chattering groups or on our own. Sometimes I stopped at the blacksmith's and, from the safety of the doorway, watched him sharpen plows. More often, I visited the town shoemaker, standing on a bench and chatting with him as he repaired boots. It was easier for me to talk to him than to my classmates.

Once we got home, we played outside if it was nice or we played school, joined by our cousin Miriam, who lived across the road. Miriam and my sister Ruth were the teachers. My sister Helen, who would start school the next year, and I were the students.

I wish I'd been as comfortable in my real school as I was in the one at home. I was the only person in Watkins who'd been crippled by polio. Did I look mysterious and tragic to the students in my first grade class? I don't know. I only know that I was very self-conscious about the brace on my right leg.

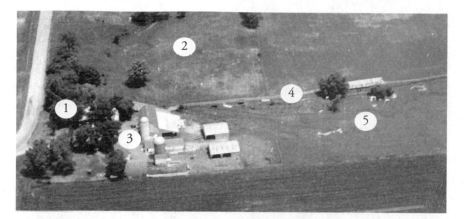

Our farm in Watkins, including (1) the farmhouse, (2) the sledding hill, (3) the new silo, (4) the tobacco shed road, and (5) the creek

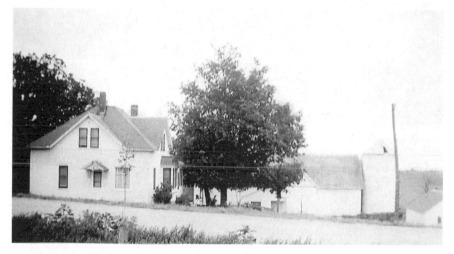

The farmhouse, barn, and old silo

My pants hid most of the metal bar that ran up the side of the lower leg and the wide leather strap that held it in place just below the knee. They didn't conceal the built-up inch-thick sole on my right shoe, though, and the metal pin that ran through it to anchor the brace. The apparatus clunked when I walked. I had to watch every step, constantly looking down to see where my weak foot was going to land.

I wanted very much to play and participate in class like other students, but I did not know how. My classmates ran around the playground, never giving a thought to their legs. I concentrated on trying to walk without a limp. They jostled and bantered with one another. I could only watch and wonder what it would feel like to be able to do that.

MEDICAL HISTORY 9-13-45
The patient has a new brace on the right leg today, which fits very nicely. Mr. Palm to try to combine the strap of the inside T strap with that of the toe check strap. Also, to have a felt metatarsal pad on the left shoe. To report to the clinic in the spring.

4-6-46
His general condition is good. No complaints to make except that it is difficult for him to walk in mud or snow. Mother states that in the past there has been a full-length steel and the last pair did not have this. She would like to have the new shoes fixed up so there is a full-length steel. ... To report in six months.

8-22-46
Patient's check strap, outside iron, and inside T strap on the right leg seem to be working satisfactorily. No further recom-

mendations, except to keep this in good repair. This boy will eventually probably have to have a triple arthrodesis. To be seen in about 4 months.

Things would be perfect, I thought, if only I didn't have to wear a brace. I felt like blaming it even when other things went wrong. Like what happened the time we made butter in class.

The farm kids brought cream to school and the town kids brought crackers and salt. The teacher poured the cream into two big jars, filling them halfway. She handed one to a student. He shook it for a while and passed it along to the next person in line.

When the jar came to me, I shook it once or twice, then it slipped out of my hands. There was a horrible crash, followed by multiple gasps. I stared in agony at the awful mess of broken glass and cream at my feet. I did not dare look up.

The teacher had us all back away so she could clean things up. There was no problem, she said. We had another jar of cream.

I thought for sure I would not get another chance to shake that one. When my turn came, though, the teacher nodded, and I took the jar. I shook it carefully and quickly passed it to the next student. Before long, we were all eating delicious homemade butter on crackers.

I was sometimes so frustrated that I misbehaved.

One afternoon, when I was being obnoxious and distracting, the teacher sent me to the coat closet in the back of the room for a time out. I crawled under a pile of coats that was heaped on the floor. That was partly to keep warm, but mostly to hide. I didn't like looking or behaving differently than others. I fell asleep.

When I awoke, the classroom was quiet. Everyone was gone, even the teacher, and so were most of the coats. The desks were clear.

I went to the door. It was locked. I looked out the window. I could see other students. They seemed to be walking home. School was out, and I was locked in.

I walked around the empty, echoing room a few times, trying to figure out how to escape. Holding my breath and hoping nobody would see me, I even opened the drawer of the teacher's desk. There was no key there, either.

I climbed up on the windowsill. I could unlock and open the window, if I wanted to. But the ground seemed a very long way down. Even if I hung on by my fingers and let go, I might get hurt.

I went back to the door. I could hear a few students at the far end of the hall. Before I could figure out what to do, however, they were gone.

Finally, after a long wait, I heard another student. I started crying loudly and banging on the door with both fists. "What's the matter?" she asked from the other side.

"I'm locked in and everybody went home," I cried.

She found a teacher, and I was soon liberated. When I got home, Mother asked why I was so late. The answer to that question was easy. It wasn't as easy to explain why I was in the coat closet in the first place. That's when I learned problems in school could lead to problems at home. I was sent to bed early that night.

Daytime frustrations affected my nights as well.

Thumping "giants" no longer tormented me. Other nightmares terrified me instead. Sometimes I dreamed there was a bad fire in the barn, in full view of the large double windows in my bedroom on the east side of the house. Sometimes logs or mud trapped my feet while I tried to run. Sometimes, for cruel variety, I would fall from a high place and wake up just before hitting the ground.

Just before I started second grade, a polio scare closed the Minnesota State Fair. The fair had been canceled before, due to the Civil War, the Dakota Indian Conflict, and World War II gas rationing, but never because of disease. That made me all the more self-conscious about my leg.

In second grade, "Ring Around the Rosy," supervised by the teachers, made way for student-organized games like "Crack the Whip," dodge ball, and tag. I knew I was not going to be able to keep up. Not even when some of the boys stomped on tin cans and clomped around with them stuck on the bottom of their shoes. I thought it strange that they had so much fun with those hunks of metal on their shoes. Then again, they could knock the cans off whenever they wanted.

I wished I could rid myself of my brace once and for all. One day, as I was struggling to untangle a knot in the brace's shoelace, I said that out loud.

"Well," said Mother, looking up from her sewing, "you know, sometime in the future you'll have an operation so you won't have to wear a brace. You won't even need a high sole on your shoe."

"When is that?" I asked eagerly.

"In a few years," she said.

I didn't remember much about my earlier operation. I just knew that having one meant going to the hospital and coming home with a scar on your foot. It would be wonderful to get rid of the brace, but "a few years" wasn't right away. I went back out to play and forgot about it.

The highlight of the second grade was getting an invitation to Granny Geislinger's house for noon lunch. My mother's mother, who had more than a dozen grandchildren at the school, lived across the street from the playground. At different times during the year she invited each of us to have a one-on-one lunch with her rather than going to the school basement for lunch. This was a very special time; when it was your turn, you had Granny's full attention.

That wasn't always the case with other people, I had discovered. Sometimes you had to do something to make them pay attention.

The school was only a block from the center of the one-block-long downtown. During recess, classmates sometimes went there to buy candy. I often tagged along. One day I walked downtown with a classmate, Augie. I gave him a quarter. I think I wanted to impress him. A quarter was a lot of money—enough to buy a ticket to a movie and a 10-cent bag of popcorn and still have a penny left over to buy a gumball Monday on the way home from school.

My mother heard about it the next afternoon when his mom visited.

"Why did you give Augie a quarter?" she asked.

"I just wanted to," I explained. "I wanted him to be my friend. He liked getting something from me."

"Money doesn't grow on trees, you know," said Mother. "If you think you can give away money, you have way too much." For a month after that, I didn't get so much as a nickel.

Like the school, the movie theater was just a few blocks from our farmhouse. When Mother and Dad gave Ruth, Helen, and me money to go to a movie, we usually walked there and back, unless the weather was bad. After a newsreel, cartoons, and previews, we would watch the main feature—Westerns with Roy Rogers, Gene Autry, and Tom Mix and comedies with the Three Stooges.

Going and coming, often in the dark, my sisters and I would study the stars. We didn't know a lot about astronomy, but we could identify the Big Dipper. We discovered that while we were watching the show the starlit sky rotated around the North Star and the Dipper turned.

Things began to turn a little for me, too. It was around this time that I made progress in making my first friend. I went to his place one afternoon, and a few weeks later, he came to mine. Mostly, we just looked around and explored. Each of our farm places was new to the other.

We both wanted BB guns. It helped my cause when I told Dad that my friend was getting one for Christmas. I got one, too, along with boxes of BBs and instructions on how to use it safely.

The piano torture began in the third grade. The lessons and practice started as a harmless activity. Mother probably assumed it would be fun. When she was in her late teens she had played piano in a local dance band in her farm neighborhood a few miles west of Watkins.

The problem was this: I hated to practice. I often dawdled at the piano in the living room for three hours before getting in my half-hour of practice. Mother kept track from the kitchen to make sure I did the full amount.

Playing marbles during recess was much more fun than playing the piano. I seem to recall losing more games than I won, but I didn't need my legs to play, so at least I had a fair chance.

I was almost in a school play that year, too. The teacher took me aside in the hall one day to explain that she had one in mind and that one of the people in it was in a wheelchair. She asked if I wanted to have that part. I told her I thought it would be interesting.

I told Mother, first thing when I got home. She listened, looking past me into the distance, but she did not say much. I could tell by the look on her face that she didn't think it was such a great idea. Finally, she said, "You better get outside to help with the chores." I never again heard about the part or even about the play itself.

8-21-48

Brace repaired, shoe built up and mailed to patient.

10-28-48

Right shoe built up and mailed to patient.

11-23-48

Right shoe built up and mailed to patient.

I didn't think much about my brace except when it broke. It always broke in the same place—at the lower end of the metal side bar, where a welded horizontal dowel went through the built-up sole just in front of the heel. There was no pain, just a snap and the sudden loss of support.

When that happened, Mother immediately sent the brace to Gillette. She also had to do that every time I got new shoes and when the steel inserted inside the shoe for stability wore out and snapped in half. If the package got to the Post Office by 1 P.M., they took it to the depot in time for the eastbound train that came through at 3. It would get to St Paul that night and be delivered to Gillette the next day. In about a week it would return, fixed and polished. In the meantime, I had to walk very carefully.

We sent shoes or my brace to Gillette 10 times between December 1946 and December 1948. I was growing rapidly. And I was active.

I might not be able to compete on the playground, but I had found a place at home to test and stretch my legs—the field road that ran east from our barn and beside an old tobacco shed. The shed had been built to dry tobacco when local farmers were experimenting with growing different crops decades earlier. A few inches of fine sand covered the road that led past it. With every rainfall, more was added, washed down from the nearby field, smoothing the surface.

I loved to run on that tobacco-shed road. When I took lunch to Dad in the field, I walked every place else, but as soon as I neared the tobacco shed I started running as fast as I could. For about a hundred feet, I ran as fast as anyone could. The four-inch-thick, hard-packed, fine sand surface allowed me to focus on going fast, not on the brace and special shoe.

All too soon, though, I was walking again. Walking and wondering about the strange things that people said sometimes. Like:

"Don't stick your tongue out. It will fall off."

"Don't cross your eyes. They'll stay that way."

"Don't go too fast; you'll hurt yourself."

"A snake is the devil. It used to have arms and legs, but then it was bad."

The words varied, but the message was clear: Bad things happen to bad people and to people who do bad things.

As I looked down at my leg, I tried to figure out what bad thing I had done. "Why ME?" I wondered. "What did I do to deserve this?"

Hours upon hours, day after day I pondered those questions. I wasn't able to come up with any good answers.

In the winter, the town kids came to our pasture hills by the dozens. They brought sleds, toboggans, skis, and even dogs. I tried skiing once, but I never got it to work. I decided I liked the toboggan better.

Our dog Rex liked it, too. He would follow me as I pulled the heavy toboggan to the top of the hill, then chase me down the hill. Sometimes he rode with me.

"I sure wish Rex could help pull that toboggan," I told Dad. "He made every trip up and down the hill with me today."

The next thing I knew, Dad and I were out in the tool shed, making a harness for Rex out of two pieces of leather from an old horse harness and two rivets. It worked wonderfully.

That wasn't the first time Rex helped me out. At dinner one night Dad sternly told me to eat my potatoes. "Think of all the hungry people in the world," he said.

"You never make Rex eat his," I reminded Dad. It was true. When we fed him the leftovers from the table, Rex always left the potatoes in his bowl. Deciding that the family dog shouldn't have privileges that I didn't, Dad never again ordered me to eat my potatoes.

It wasn't quite as easy as that to get out of my piano lessons. Quitting was not an option. A recital was only a few weeks away. My teacher told me I could pick any song in my practice book for my piece. I decided I liked "Home on the Range" the best. Then I found out that I had to play the whole thing by heart, with no sheet music in front of me. It was scary, but I thought if others could do it, I could, too. The recital went well, but after it was over, I raised such a fuss that Mother and Dad reluctantly allowed me to stop taking lessons.

I tried roller-skating at the skating rink in Kimball, a town a few miles away. Many of my classmates went there on Sunday afternoons. The rented skates kept falling off. I ended up sitting alone on the floor, an abject failure, struggling to get the clamps and straps to stay on my right shoe while all around me others were having fun, laughing and skating around in a circle, and chasing or holding on to each other. I was not much interested in skating after that.

We were all interested, however, when the old silo had to come down. That didn't happen every day; it was more like once in a lifetime.

Dad explained what was going to happen: Our tractor was going to pull the silo over while a crane guided it and gently lowered it to the ground. It had to fall just right, between the barn and the hen house. The granary across from the hen house was in slight danger, but not the pig barn down the hill.

While Mother kept children out of harm's way, Dad and the crane operator wrapped the wooden structure with cables. They checked the setup from every angle.

"Bring the tractor and back it in here," Dad yelled to me. I was only 10, but like a lot of farm kids I drove tractor all the time.

I backed up to where Dad was standing. He was holding a hitch pin and the end of one of the cables that was wrapped around the silo. At a slight wave of his finger, I stopped. He dropped the pin into the clevis, connecting the cable to the tractor. Then he backed away.

Sitting on the tractor, pushing a brake with each foot, I held the machine motionless. I expected that any moment Dad would climb up one side of the tractor and I'd be sent to a safer spot near the house, "in case something happened."

Dad looked at the silo and the crane operator. They double-checked everything, nodded, and then waved to each other. They were ready.

"Is it in first?" Dad yelled.

I looked down at the shift lever between my legs and nodded. It was.

Dad began circling his arm, signaling me to nudge the hand clutch a little and start inching forward. The tractor wheels gripped the ground. The cable slowly tightened. I watched him closely. Any second now, he would motion me to stop, have me set the brakes, and let him drive.

Instead, Dad motioned to keep going. Suddenly I realized that the silo was coming down. That I was pulling it down. As I did so, Dad moved around, watching everything, nodding to the crane operator.

We stood there afterwards, admiring our work. We'd laid it right where we wanted it to be.

Finally I looked up at Dad and asked, "What do we do with it now?" I was already imagining what a great bonfire it would make.

That's when Dad explained that my next job was to salvage the good boards from the building. I was going to pull out every nail, with a hammer, put them on the hay wagon, and haul them to the tobacco shed for storage. I would haul the bad boards to the pasture beyond the tobacco shed, where they'd be burned. It took weeks to get that done.

We were not allowed to climb other buildings because we might damage their roof shingles, but we could climb the new silo. It was the tallest building on the farm, taller even than the barn. It had vertical concrete ribs that held horizontal steel hoops a few inches out from the wall. The hoops were about 15 inches apart. It was easy to reach from one to the next on the way up. The thing was like one huge climbing wall.

The only rule Mother and Dad set was this: "Don't climb so high that you can't get down." I never did. With strong arms and my good left leg, I climbed it often.

3-19-49

There is about 3/4 of an inch discrepancy leg length and after foot stabilization is done, this will probably be about 1 inch or more. The boy is now 10 years old. Certainly when he is no more than 12 years old consideration should be given for foot stabilization procedure probably of the Lambrinudi type. An epiphyseal arrest the distal end of the left femur can be done at that time.

That summer I noticed how tadpoles became frogs. Rex wouldn't miss a trek along the creek for anything. He even helped me catch frogs. He seemed to be able to tell what I was trying to do.

We also got a call that summer from Gillette, or rather my Aunt Clara, across the road, did. We didn't have a phone at our farm until much later, when I was in high school. Dad drove uptown to the telephone office to return the call. I never heard what it was about and I never asked. I assumed it had something to do with my brace.

I was now a fifth grader. Sister Caroline, my teacher, was making it my best year in school so far. I was also part of a loose-knit group of friends. When a classmate put together an order for fireworks, I was one of the boys he invited to join him. I put $3 into the kitty. The fireworks arrived by train, and we distributed them in school. I used my firecrackers at home, but they were fairly common and my parents never knew exactly where I got them.

I was feeling almost normal in fact. My right leg was shorter than my left, but my left leg was very strong and perfectly healthy. For jumping, hopping and climbing, it was like a leg and a half.

Late in December, my parents told me that we had an appointment at Gillette on Thursday, January 5, 1950. The doctors wanted to see if I was ready for the operation that would enable me to get rid of my brace.

The day before the examination, after I got home from school, Mother mentioned that the doctors might want me to stay at the hospital for the operation rather than coming home right away.

I looked down at the metal attached to my leg, then back up at her. I didn't know what to say. I couldn't remember much from the last time I was in Gillette, but the operation I got at age 5 didn't hurt anymore. If another one could fix my foot, I was ready to spend a few months in the hospital. I would do anything to get rid of my brace and wear regular shoes.

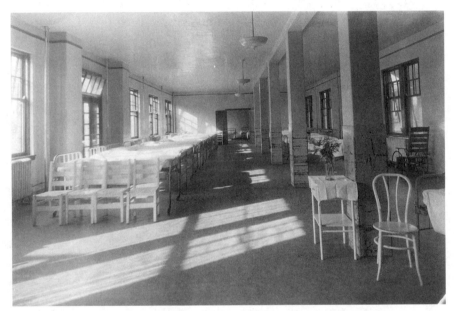

Ward 6, the older boys' ward, where I spent several years of my childhood

*W*e had a quick breakfast the next day and were on the road to St. Paul by six. The Twin Cities had received five inches of snow during the preceding three days and the temperature was well below freezing. That wasn't unusual, not for January in Minnesota. What was unusual was that Dad was with Mother and me, instead of at home. He'd arranged with a neighbor to milk our cows—we had 20 head of Holsteins—and feed them and the other animals.

On the way, Mother and Dad told me again that the doctor might say it was time for an operation. I peeked at the scar on my heel, trying to remember the previous one. I couldn't. It couldn't have been a big deal, I figured. If it meant getting rid of the brace and special shoe, I was ready.

The route to Gillette was a familiar one. We went the same way every time I needed a checkup. I had the towns along Highway 55 memorized: Watkins, Kimball, South Haven, Annandale, Maple Lake, Buffalo, Rockford, Medina, New Hope, and Robbinsdale. Then we were in the Twin Cities, halfway there. Another hour of city driving would get us to 1003 Ivy Avenue East in St. Paul, where Gillette was located.

We typically entered the Gillette outpatient department by eight, waited while the doctors took care of the morning's operations, ate a bag lunch, waited some more, then saw a doctor and returned home, stopping in Medina at the Eat and Run Café. We especially liked the banana cream pies they made there.

This trip was different, however. By nine we were checked in and sitting on a bench in Gillette's new outpatient wing. The bench looked like a church pew and it seemed as long as the barn back home.

"You're Lorrayne Maus?" a nurse said, approaching Mother.

"Yes," Mother responded.

The nurse bent toward me. "Well, hi, Mickey. I'm so happy to see you again. You probably don't even remember me." She chatted for a moment with Mother, then rushed off.

Someone remembered me, even after five years! She was right, though. I didn't remember her. There was a lot that I didn't recall, it seemed. That was a little scary.

"Was I ever called Mickey?" I asked Mother. It was intriguing to think that someone had known me well enough to give me a nickname, especially one connected to a character as popular as Mickey Mouse.

"The nurses must have called you Mickey, I suppose," she replied. She looked past me into the distance, frustrated, I think, at not knowing something so basic about my childhood. Wondering, maybe, what else she and Dad had missed out on during the three months I had been at the hospital last time.

After two hours, another nurse directed us to an examining area with curtains around it. I removed my shoes, socks, and clothes, put on the white hospital gown that the nurse handed me, and sat on the padded oak examining table. My parents sat in a pair of chairs nearby. We waited another hour. They seemed comfortable, but I could not help fidgeting.

Finally, the nurse poked her head in and announced, "Here they come."

She pulled back the curtain, and Doctor Frank Babb and an entourage of eight white-clothed staff members approached the table. One of the aides picked up my chart from the chair at the end of the table and

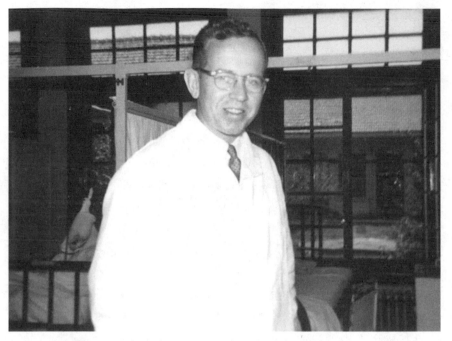

Dr. Frank Babb, my orthopedic surgeon. Photo by John Andrisen

handed it to Dr. Babb. While all the others quietly watched, he quickly read a few notes, flipped a few pages, then handed the chart back.

There was no doubt about who was in charge. Everyone was watching Dr. Babb—the staff nurse, the scheduling secretary, the physiotherapist, the stenographer, the resident, and some interns, as well as Mother, Dad, and me.

He nodded a greeting to my parents. Next, he turned to me. In one breath, he said, "Hi, Richard," and "You are Richard, aren't you?" He didn't seem to expect an answer.

He turned to his staff and talked to them for a minute, using words and sentences I did not understand. I watched and listened to him carefully. I didn't know who he was really, but he appeared to be in charge of my life, my destiny.

With his left hand on my right knee, he held the fingers of his right hand above my right toes. "Can you lift your toes to touch my fingers?" he asked.

"No," I responded, trying anyway.

"Can you lift your foot to touch my fingers?" he asked.

"No," I answered again. I wanted to add, "I can wiggle my ears, though." Why didn't he ask for something I could do, rather than the one thing I couldn't?

He next measured my legs from hip to ankle, using a tape measure. He turned to a staff person and said something about next week. Then he said something to Mother about next week. She looked at Dad and nodded. Without saying anything to me, the doctor and staff left, off to see the patient at the next table.

"You mean we have to come back next week?" I asked.

Mother, talking slowly but firmly, said, "They want you to stay here. The operation will be next week."

Dad quickly added, "After that you won't need the brace anymore."

"How long will I have to stay?" I asked.

"A month or two," Mother answered. "But, don't worry. We will come to visit on the day of the operation and every second Sunday afternoon after that."

MEDICAL RECORD 1-5-50

To be re-admitted. The patient has residual poliomyelitis involving the right lower extremity with 1-1/2 inches of shortening on this side. He has a fairly good quadriceps and hamstrings and very good power in the calf muscles, but he has no anterior tibial or peroneal power at all, nor can I make out any power in his posterior tibial, this may just be weak. He should have a stabilization of his right foot, probably a Lambrinudi operation as recommended by Dr. Goldner, and, at some later date, an epiphyseal arrest at the left knee. There is no evidence of scoliosis as yet, but he does have a rather tight iliotibial band on the right which should be observed further while in the hospital. Dr. Babb.

Someone else needed the examining area. Barefoot and clutching the hospital gown to make sure it stayed closed where it needed to, I returned to the long bench in the waiting area. As we sat down to await instructions, another group of smiling nurses came by. "Hi, Mickey." "So glad to see you again."

A terrible noise emerged from a small room in front of us. I thought at first that it was a worker with an electric tool. We knew that a doctor, a nurse, and a young boy were in there. We had seen them go in. The noise started and stopped in an unpredictable pattern. It was earsplitting. Then we heard the boy. What were they doing to make him scream so loudly?

Mother fidgeted. She looked as if she wished we were somewhere else. The noise kept starting and stopping; the boy kept yelling. Mother rubbed her hands together as she always did when she was nervous. She finally suggested we move to the other end of the long bench, where it might not be as noisy.

Eventually a nurse arrived with a wheelchair. She motioned for me to get in. I thought that was odd. I had walked into the hospital by myself, without any help. On the other hand, I didn't have on shoes anymore or clothes. I got in without arguing. She pushed me down a long hall, past a new, not quite finished game room, to the elevator. We went up one floor, along another long hall, and then stopped.

Mother put the bag with my clothes in it on my lap. She kissed me on the forehead, while Dad patted my shoulder. They said "Goodbye," and the nurse rolled me away.

That was when it hit me. They were going home. I wasn't, at least not yet. The tears rolled down my face, and my body shook. I cried as I had never cried. I also felt more alone than ever before.

The nurse turned left at the end of a bare hall and down a hall with glass-enclosed rooms on either side. Inside I could see beds filled with other children. Halfway down, we passed the nurses' desk. The hospital had a peculiar smell, not like anything at home, not even in the barn. It made me almost throw up.

My room was at the far end, on the left. I was in the hospital's newest wing, located above the outpatient department. The room had two beds, which could be separated by a curtain. Mine was the first one, just inside the door. The other one, which was empty, was next to a window with a view of part of the hospital—the operating room, I discovered later—and of the wooded grounds. There was a closet and an adjoining bathroom.

The nurse instructed me to climb onto the bed. She immediately left with the wheelchair and my clothes. She returned with a white diaper, with strings at each corner. She told me to put it on under my hospital gown.

"Why do I need to wear that?" I asked.

"Everybody has to wear them," she responded.

I had stopped crying by that time. I needed to watch the activity in my end of the ward, I decided. I needed to figure out what was going on. It shouldn't be hard to do. There was nothing to distract me, no radio, nothing to read, no toys.

Dinner came on a tray. At home, I only got food on a tray when I was very sick. I was not sick. But I was in a hospital. This is what a hospital is like, I thought.

The rooms across the hall had nurses going in and out all the time. I could hear crying and moaning in some of them. My room was quiet and bare. A nurse came to turn off the lights for bedtime. Afterwards, there was still an orange glow, from nightlights in the room and hall.

It felt weird, lying there in that dim orange light. I wondered: How long would it take me to walk home? I was not quite 11, but I knew every turn in the road from Gillette to Watkins. I couldn't get lost. I gave up on the idea when I realized I had no clothes and no idea where they were being kept.

The next few days were pretty much the same. I sat on my bed all day, in a hospital gown and diaper, keeping an eye on the activity in the hallway outside my room. If I were at home, I thought, I would be in school. School! I hadn't had a chance to say goodbye to anyone, since I didn't know they would want to keep me here. Did any of my classmates wonder where I was or what was happening to me?

On Monday, someone came by with a library cart. I did not want a book. I wasn't in the mood to read, and I didn't know what kind to ask for, in any case. She left one anyway. I didn't read it. If I was going to figure out what was going on, to get the lay of the land, I couldn't afford to miss anything that moved, anything that made a sound.

I had plenty of time to study my surroundings. Everything looked familiar except the fat brown rubber cord hanging on the wall by my bed. My eyes kept going back to it. What was it for? Was it a tube, or was it a wire? One end of it went into the wall. I had never seen anything like it before. It was the most peculiar thing in the room.

Finally, I had to touch it, turn it, hold it. Looking at it for days and from every angle had not helped me understand it. I lifted one end from the hook holding it onto the wall and looked closer. I was ready, if I heard the footsteps of a nurse, to quickly place it back. I didn't want to get into trouble for fiddling with it.

The cord had a little piece of hard rubber about the size of a pencil eraser sticking out the end of it. Around that there was a ring that was loose and wiggly. I fiddled, wiggled, poked, and pushed—until one time the thing on the end stayed in.

What should I do now? How could I get it back out? What if the nurse found out I had jammed it?

I hung the cord back on the hook and sat in the middle of the bed, pretending nothing happened.

Almost before I recognized her footsteps, the nurse was there, asking, "Did you want something?"

"No," I quickly answered.

She was holding the brown cord. She told me not to push the button if I did not want anything. It made a light go on at her desk. She also showed me how pressing the ring made the button pop back out.

I decided then and there: Nurses were hard to fool. Just like my parents.

With nothing left to explore, my mind turned to lonelier, scarier thoughts. I knew people sometimes died in hospitals. Would one of the patients across the hall die? Would I see them take the body out of the room? Did they sneak the dead bodies out? Did they tell anybody?

I wasn't so much worried about myself. After all, I had not been in a bad accident or anything. I was simply having an operation to fix my foot. I didn't have to worry. I had had one operation already and come through fine. This one, the last one I would ever have to have, would be no different.

Monday was interesting for another reason. In the afternoon, a nurse came in to tell me that I would be getting a roommate the next day, a boy, 16. He would be coming in from surgery. There might be nurses coming in and going out for a few days, and there would be more lights and distractions.

It wouldn't be a bother, I told her. Any activity would be more interesting than quiet, lonely boredom, I thought to myself. It would be nice to have someone to talk with.

On Tuesday I ate lunch quickly. I wanted to be ready when they brought the boy in from surgery. I didn't want to miss a thing.

At about one o'clock a cart arrived, pushed by two nurses wearing white masks. I could not have been more alert. I sat on my bed, watching the activity, analyzing it.

The boy had a cast on one of his legs, which was resting on three pillows. His toes were orange. I watched as three more nurses came to help move him onto his bed.

Later, when the nurses were gone, he started moaning. Then he was quiet again. Then he threw up and moaned with pain again. The nurses came by regularly to check on him that night and all the next day. The vomiting lasted only a few hours, but the moaning continued all night.

He was not very good company. He didn't say much to anyone. He was sick and hurting. I had never seen anyone that sick before. He must have fallen off a silo or something, I thought. Maybe a car or a train hit him. I was sure glad that I was not having surgery.

The next day, a mop lady came to clean the floor on my side of the room.

"I wonder what happened to him," I said, as she mopped under my bed.

"I think he had an operation yesterday," she said.

An operation? My mind raced. Surgery and an operation were the same thing?

Suddenly things looked very different. He had had what I was going to have. When I watched him moaning and vomiting, I was looking at myself in a few days. This was so much worse than I had envisioned.

I crawled under the covers. I cried. I wondered again where my clothes were. Even if I got lost running home, that would be better than this.

On Thursday, a week after I was admitted, Dr. Babb and the white-robed staff came again. He took a quick look at my legs and said I was ready for surgery, next Monday. Then they left.

In the afternoon, I heard something new. It wasn't one of the carts that routinely creaked across the cracks in the floor. I knew that sound. This cart tinkled as it went. When it came to my room, I discovered why. It had rows and rows of glass test tubes and glass slides in metal racks with holes.

The person who was pushing the cart stopped at my bed. Before I could say anything, she took my hand in hers—and pricked my finger with something sharp! I flinched and tried to pull away. The worst was already over, she explained. She squeezed a few drops of blood from my finger onto a glass slide, smiled, said a few words, and before I could say "blood test," she was gone.

Early Sunday evening, I rejected the notion of trying to escape. I decided, after a great deal of thought, that the important thing was to get rid of the brace, whatever it took.

Then the nurses came to get me ready for surgery. The first one was carrying an empty one-gallon can with a rubber tube connected to it.

"Did you ever have an enema?" she asked.

"A what?" I answered.

It was standard for all surgeries, she said. She explained what she intended to do. She would fill the can with warm soapy water, push the end of the tube into my butt, hold the can high, and let the water run into my body. After that, I needed to be ready to run for the toilet. The water would make my body try to get rid of everything in my intestines.

"Don't just tell me if it hurts," she said. "Only tell me if it hurts so badly you can't stand any more."

After I sat on the toilet for an hour or so and emptied myself out, she started filling the huge tub in the bathroom. At home, we only put a few inches of water in the tub, which was a much smaller, normal size. Here the tub was filled almost to the top with wonderful, warm water, and when I got out I was allowed to use two towels.

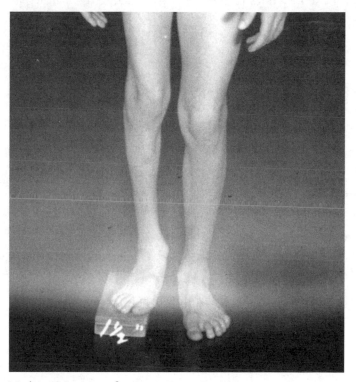

My legs in January of 1950

Another nurse came into the room about eight. She had a small cart and wanted to "prep" me.

"Does it hurt much?" I ask.

"No, not at all," she said. "We just shave your leg and wrap it up."

I had often seen Dad shave, but never a leg. She was right. It did not hurt.

When she was done with the right leg, she indicated that she needed the left one.

"What for?" I asked.

"I have to do both of them," she said.

"But my left leg doesn't need it," I protested. "My right leg is having the operation."

"It says here that the left knee needs prep, too," she insisted.

I tried to push her hand away. I could do everything with my left leg. Hop, skip, jump. Lift anything. Nobody my age had a better left leg. There simply was no problem with the left leg. It had to be a mistake.

She tried again, and again I resisted. She left the room and came back with another nurse, a big one, with a black stripe on her white hat.

"We need to prep your left knee, Richard," she said. "Dr. Babb said so right here." She showed the written order to me, but not long enough for me to be able to read it.

I knew what she wanted to do. I knew that it did not hurt. I just could not understand why they needed to operate on my perfectly good left leg.

Most of all, though, I was thinking about the boy lying next to me. The operation he had had, on just one leg, had made him very sick. It still hurt a lot. It was beginning to look like mine could be twice as bad.

I thought of nothing else for the remainder of a very restless night.

Monday morning arrived, and I discovered that I could not have breakfast.

"How about a drink of water?" I asked.

"Nope," they said. "Not until after surgery."

After awhile, a pair of nurses with masks came to get me. I had to wait in the cold hallway before they wheeled me into an even colder operating room. When I shivered and complained, they gave me a little blanket.

They lifted me onto a large metal table. There was a huge light above it, but it wasn't turned on yet. "Might be warmer if it was," I thought. A nurse taped my right arm down to the table. She inserted the biggest needle I ever saw into a vein there, taped the needle onto the arm, and connected it to a plastic tube. After that, she reached for another needle, even bigger. Before I could panic, she stuck it in the tube connected to the first needle. She asked me what town I was from. As I started to answer, I felt something cold moving through my arm . . .

The next instant, I was back in my room, throwing up.

The pain was not as bad as I had imagined it would be. The routine was about what I expected, though, from watching my roommate: Wake up, vomit, and go back to sleep; wake up, vomit, etc. I went through that about a dozen times. Then the pain arrived. The codeine they gave me helped, but it made me sleepy. After about five days, the pain eased and they could switch to aspirin.

I saw my parents after the operation, I know, but I barely remember them being there. They could not stay long that day; they had to get back for chores. They came back six days later, on Sunday afternoon. It was good to see them.

1-16-50

ANESTHETIC: Pentothal-curare, nitrous oxide

DURATION OF OPERATION   Began: 11:25 A.M. Ended
1:45 P.M.

DESCRIPTION OF OPERATION: The foot, ankle and leg were
prepared and draped in a sterile manner and a pneumatic
tourniquet was applied. A straight horizontal incision was
made over the lateral aspect of the right foot. The areolar tissue was removed from the sinus tarsi. With a wide chisel the
head of the astragalus was removed together with a wedge
from the inferior body of the astragalus. The cartilage was
removed from the remainder of the talonavicular joint, from
the calcaneocuboid joint and from the talocalcaneal joint. The
opposing raw bone surfaces were then fitted together and held
with three wire staples. Cancellous bone which had been
removed was packed between the opposing bone surfaces. The
skin was closed and a long leg plaster cast was applied with the
knee in moderate flexion. Immediate postoperative condition
was good.

OPERATOR: F.S. Babb, M.D.

   The orthopedic surgeon had put three staples in my right foot to prevent it from curling and rolling. He had also put staples on both sides of
my left leg, just above the knee, at the growth plate. That would prevent
the left femur from growing while the right leg caught up in length. My
right leg was encased in plaster, my left in a bandage that kept it immo-
bile but slightly flexed. Until they were removed, I wouldn't be able to
roll over in bed. I'd have to sleep on my back.

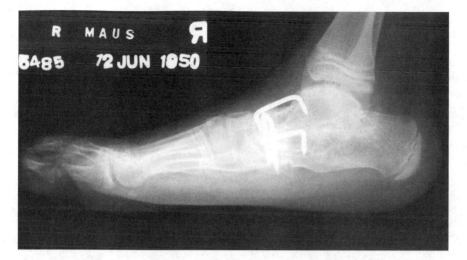

X-ray, 6-12-50, showing staples inserted to stabilize right foot

In 10 days, I got a new cast on the right leg. When they took the old one off, I discovered the source of the terrible sound I had heard in the outpatient department on the day I had come to Gillette. It was the sound the vibrating cast cutter made when it cut through plaster. The doctor showed me how it worked, though, so I didn't react in the hysterical way the boy had on the day I was admitted.

1-26-50

X-ray of the left knee of January 23 shows the distal end of the femur to be stapled in the usual manner. The staples on the medial side are a little too low and this knee should be watched for a knock-knee deformity. Post operative x-rays of the right foot show the foot following Lambrinudi to be in only a fair posi-

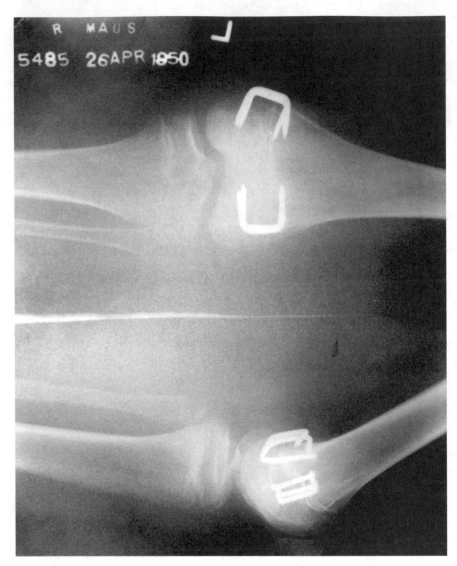

X-rays, 4-26-50: showing staples inserted on either side of left leg to keep the growth plate from expanding

tion. A little too much of the navicular bone has been removed, and the foot has been flattened considerably. At the next change of plaster, an attempt should be made to try to restore the lateral arch to prevent a rocker bottom foot . . . Dr. Babb

Two weeks after my operation, they transferred me to Ward 6. There were 26 guys there. Most were up and around on crutches or, like me, in wheelchairs. A few were confined to bed. At 10, I was one of the youngest patients. They usually ranged in age from 12 to 21.

At the front of the ward, on the left, was, literally, a "bathroom"—a place to give baths. Bed patients were wheeled in there on carts to get sponge baths and an occasional hair wash. Next to that was an open area with tables and chairs where "up" patients could eat and, later, watch TV. The nurse's station was beyond that and then the big double doors to the outside.

On the right at the front were a few cubicles for bed patients, storage rooms, and a large restroom. In the back was a room with about 10 beds that was usually reserved for the older boys. The rest of us filled the beds that occupied the remainder of the ward.

At the beginning of February, they sent me to Gillette's school, a newer west wing called "Michael J. Dowling Memorial Hall." I needed help getting my chair up the ramp at the beginning of the school hallway. A bigger boy on crutches with one good leg helped me with a push.

The auditorium was there. I recognized it right away. It was where I had watched cartoons in bed after my first operation when I was 5. There were also classrooms and a library.

One of the three morning classes was a math class. The room was crowded; there were about eight wheelchairs, as well as 10 desks for walkers or those with crutches. Nearly everyone in the class was in a different grade and using a different book. When you first arrived, the teacher found a page that you thought you could do and made that your first assignment. You couldn't expect much help. By the time everyone was arranged and seated and the books passed out, it was often time to put everything away and roll to the next class.

I got a fever a few days later. They transferred me back to the new admitting unit, where I had my own room again. After six days, on the day before Valentine's Day, they sent me back to Ward 6.

The doctor removed the bandage on my left leg on February 16, a month after the operation. My leg smelled the way toes do after they haven't been washed for a few days. I had to be very careful when I scratched it in order not to tear the sensitive skin.

It was good to be able to take an almost normal bath again, in a tub with the casted right leg on a bench to keep it from getting wet. About that time, though, they discovered that I couldn't straighten my left leg fully. It hurt too much. Doctors and nurses tried many painful times over the next month to get it to extend all the way, but with no success.

Finally, the third week in March they took me to the operating room, put me nearly to sleep, forced my left leg straight, and put a cast on it, one that stretched from the upper ankle to the upper thigh. At the same time, they replaced the cast on my right leg, giving me one that had a rubber heel on the foot so I could walk on it.

I had casts on both legs, but I could walk without crutches. On the ward, I helped one of my friends build a model car and mastered the yo-yo with another one. I also went back to school.

One day I got out of the standard naptime by going with a man to a room where he asked me a lot of questions. It was a test, but an interesting one, unlike usual school tests. I was just glad he didn't have a needle.

3-24-1950
PSYCHOLOGICAL REPORT
COUNTY Ramsey
Handicaps none for testing
Test used Stanford-Binet

Summary
Richard took an immediate interest in the test and appeared to
be enthusiastic and alert in his responses. Basal age is nine
years with tests passed through the fourteen year level.
Abstract verbal and concrete-performance ability are developing about evenly. In addition, Richard shows a rather highly
developed social sense on items which require insight into
absurd situations – actions and speech also indicate better than
average social intelligence. His over-all IQ is that of a person
with normal intelligence.

They removed the left cast again in late April. After a few days, I once
again could not straighten the leg. In May they took me back to the OR,
put me to sleep again, and put another ankle-to-thigh cast on it.

When the right leg cast was finally removed, I started walking in
shoes again. I didn't need a brace anymore, but I did need a built-up
inch-and-one-half-thick sole on the right foot. They took off the left cast
in late May, but they saved the back half of the plaster so it could be
used as a night splint.

On June 17, 1950, I was judged ready to go home. The month or two
that Mother had predicted I'd have to spend in the hospital had turned
into six. School was out by the time I returned.

I spent the summer tearing around the farm, getting to know my sisters and brother again and roaming the fields with Rex. I didn't give a second thought to what the fall might hold. Things had taken longer than expected, but the worst was behind me, now that I'd had my operation. From now on, everything would be different, better.

By the time I started sixth grade, I had not seen my classmates for eight months. I knew everyone's name, though. After all, our school had only one class in every grade. They knew my name, too.

But they had changed. Some were bigger, taller. Some had different friends than they'd had the year before. I wasn't anybody's friend. Nobody even said, "Oh, you're back." They'd learned to get along without me.

At noon recess the first day, two team leaders quickly chose sides for a game of baseball. I was afraid they would choose me last, but, actually, nobody chose me at all. Before they finished picking, they ran off to start the game.

Couldn't they even see me? I almost cried. Instead I asked a nearby classmate, "Which side am I on?"

"Our side," he answered. Maybe he figured an extra player couldn't hurt his team, or maybe he didn't really count me.

The rest of school, that day and for the rest of the year, went about the same as recess, even though the brace was gone. I felt like I was invisible except when I was doing something stupid or embarrassing.

My left leg was doing quite well, but I still had trouble with my right foot. It tended to drop, hanging down in front. The following spring the doctor told us that I needed another operation. I was to report back to Gillette once school was out.

CHAPTER 4

*b*efore I returned to Gillette, my brother Phil and I spent a whole
warm afternoon riding inner tubes down the creek. We explored
all the way across our farm—from the sliding hill north of the
house, past the barn and tobacco shed, and south to the railroad tracks.
In some places, the water was waist deep with a sandy bottom. In other
places, the creek was fast moving and shallow with tall grass and a
muddy bottom. It was a real adventure for us and for Rex and lots of
fun. Without my old leather and metal brace, I could go almost anywhere.

Phil and I never talked about polio, my foot, or the hospital. Because
the rules about visiting were so restrictive, he'd never visited me at
Gillette. None of my siblings had. I never discussed what happened there
with them—or with anybody else, for that matter.

On July 10, 1951, I was back in Ward 6. As usual, the operation I was
scheduled for wouldn't take place for another week. In the meantime, I
reacquainted myself with the place and the people.

I had left the ward over a year earlier, but I felt right at home. I knew
the routine. I knew all the nurses and aides. Some patients were new,
worried and scared, but there were a lot of familiar faces, too. Some, like
me, had been home and were now back. A couple of friends, Dennis and
Walter, had never left.

Dennis had had a spinal fusion and a series of body casts. His arms were strong, but his torso and legs were paralyzed. At least he could now roll over and sit up, using the trapeze bar attached to the bed above him. He was a few years older than I was. He had a radio and an endless supply of jokes picked up from radio DJs. He seemed to know everyone's favorite songs.

Walter had been badly burned. He was undergoing a seemingly endless series of skin grafts that tied him up in knots. To transfer good skin from his thigh to his burned arm, for example, they put him in a cast that held the thigh and arm together for many weeks until the skin "took" and transferred to the new surface. Then he would go back to surgery for another graft. Most of his face and neck was scar tissue. It was painful and hard for him to move. He was about my age, 12, and a great chess player. His home was nearby in St. Paul, and on the weekends he had many visitors.

The ward was a huge bedroom and playroom combined. At any given time, about half of the patients were doing something on their own— sleeping, reading, watching others, trying to poke something down an itchy cast, or listening to a rare radio. Others, in small groups around the ward, were playing chess, arm wrestling, playing hearts, or watching TV. On nice summer days, many of the beds were rolled outside to give the patients a few hours of warm sunshine.

Nurses and aides were seemingly all over the place, all the time. Staff members from other parts of the hospital were also in and out throughout the day. Therapists, doctors, the barber, the librarian, laundry and cleaning people and, sometimes, volunteers passed through or came to see a patient or take one somewhere else.

The wide range of ages in the ward had its effect. The older boys generally dominated the play areas and sometimes tormented the younger ones. Some of the older kids were outright mean, and others were protective.

Occasionally there were fights. There was an unwritten rule, though: You couldn't attack someone's handicapped area. It was not fair to take advantage of an opponent's weak spots or make an injury or disability worse.

There was also a bond. We had something in common. We were all handicapped and away from home.

Generally, it was easy to get along with most of the patients in the ward and easy to get to know them. Since I was still walking quite nicely during that first week, I could help those in wheelchairs. If someone in bed dropped something out of reach on the floor, I could get it for him and strike up a conversation.

We found ways to entertain ourselves. Two bed-ridden patients on opposite sides of the long aisle played catch with a tennis ball. Whenever the ball got out-of-hand, there was a mad scramble, just like the race to get a fly ball in the stands at a ballpark. After a game of "Keep Away," someone would return the ball to the original owners and the sequence would begin again.

There was also school, even though it was July. In the summer, most classes were reading classes. We could read anything we wanted.

The library was my favorite place in the school wing of Gillette. Mrs. Hughes, the librarian, was a very nice woman. She liked to collect and sort stamps, but I couldn't get interested in it. She knew every book in the library and its location. She helped me find the ones I liked. They were mostly about airplanes, books filled with pictures of P-51 Mustang fighter planes and B-24 Liberator bombers from World War II, which had ended just a few years before. To my mind, flying and tumbling about in the sky were the perfect antidotes to being confined to a bed.

I also read *Kon-Tiki* and other grand adventures, including many of the Jules Verne books, such as *Twenty Thousand Leagues Under the Sea.* His *Journey to the Moon and Back* fit right in with a movie I had seen in Watkins called *Destination Moon.* Yes, I thought. We'll get to the moon and that is how.

The library was also a very quiet place, unlike the ward. There might be girls from Ward 8 there, but, as in class, we weren't allowed to talk to each other. Socializing of any kind was not permitted.

The teachers at the hospital always seemed more like aides or substitutes. The teachers at home stood in front of a class of 30 students and asked questions, explained things, and often wrote on the blackboard. At Gillette the teacher usually sat at her desk unless she had to walk across the room to help somebody with a lesson or to help someone get comfortable.

It was nearly impossible to study subjects together—everyone in the classroom came from a different school. Most of us didn't know what we were studying at home, what books we were using, and where we were in them.

For that matter, it was summer. I shouldn't have to go to school at all, I thought. I should be on vacation.

The teachers at the hospital always mailed a report card home after I was discharged. My grades were usually D's. They reflected my attitude more than anything else. They never gave any indication of what I studied or how much I learned.

On Monday, July 16, I was transferred to Ward 1, given another enema, and prepared for surgery on Tuesday.

To solve the foot drop problem, Dr. Babb was going to remove a piece of bone from the lower part of my right leg and insert it into the rear of the anklebones so that the foot and leg would fuse as one bone. The foot would be fused at a right angle to the leg, eliminating the foot drop.

The trip to the operating room held no surprises. I knew what to expect now. I was not scared, but I knew it was going to hurt and where. I comforted myself with the thought that it might not be as bad as before, since they were only operating on one leg this time.

7-17-51

Operation began: 11:00 A.M.

DESCRIPTION OF OPERATION: A four-inch vertical incision was made on the posterior aspect of the right leg extending from the calf down to the heel ... It was decided to make vertical groove into the calcaneus to receive the bone block, and this was performed. Then attention was turned to the tibia about two inches above the epiphyseal line where a 1-1/2 x 1 centimeter square was removed by the use of a handchuck with a small drill point followed by an osteotome and hammer. This piece of bone was then placed in the vertical groove fashioned in the calcaneus ... A plaster cast was applied from the toes to the vicinity of the tibial tuberosity with the foot held at 90°. ... The patient withstood the procedure well and left the operating room in good condition. F.S. Babb M.D.

Operation ended: 12:25 P.M.

I was looking forward to my first "rollover" long before I got off the pain-killing medications. Lying on my back for over a week had caused other aches, including sore "sheet-rash" elbows, a common problem for patients stuck in one position. Even if rolling over caused more leg pain, it felt so refreshing to the rest of the body.

The next step was the removal of the surgery stitches. If the cast covering the stitches was not to be replaced and was small, it was removed in the ward. Otherwise, a trip to the cast room near the OR was necessary.

Because the resident doctor or intern removing the stitches was usually new, he always acted as if it was my first time also. After watching him tentatively clip and pull a few stitches, I always had the overwhelming urge to ask him to let me do it. I never actually asked and they never offered. Watching him, though, I thought that I could be an orthopedic surgeon.

Once I was up in a wheelchair, there was so much more to do. Racing from one end of the ward to the other was fun, though the nurses didn't tolerate it well. We had to wait until they were either gone or busy. By the time they caught the wheelchairs, the race usually had a winner. Anyone who coasted down the laundry cart ramp outside Ward 6 or got hurt in a race got the rest of the day back in bed and a lecture about not being ready for a wheelchair.

About once a week, volunteers took us to the playroom downstairs in the new admitting unit. It was well equipped with table and floor shuffleboards, dartboards, and game tables. It was something different to do, but we were with the same few patients as in the ward or classrooms. If the girls from Ward 8 were there, they were kept at the other end of the room from us.

A cooking class made school more interesting. We made five recipes. I had helped with meals at home—peeling vegetables, popping popcorn, wiping the plates after dinner—but I had never been responsible for a dish from start to finish. I got an incredible sense of accomplishment when I made apple crunch (see page 167) all by myself with only a few tips from the instructor.

The ward was filled with memorable people, too. The usually hyper-busy head nurse, Miss Hennesy, would linger by your bed and talk, someone told me—if you asked her about pheasant hunting. She was so tiny; it seemed like the kick of a shotgun would knock her over. When I told her that, she replied that she used a smaller gauge gun, a .410.

Miss Hennesy was usually in a rush, barking orders to staff and patients. She also loved to whack the foot of the bed as she passed, to jar it enough to move it in line with the others. On those rare occasions when she came around and offered an alcohol or lotion backrub, you knew everything was in order.

Mrs. Beaver, on the other hand, was calm, steady, and very tolerant. You knew it would be a pleasant day if she were the head nurse.

My favorite staff person was an aide named Mrs. Berndt. She had such a nice smile. She would do anything for anybody. While she was on duty, nobody ever spilled a glass of water in a bed on a dare.

Mrs. Berndt's own boys were finished with school and away from home. I sometimes wished she were my mother. She was there. Mother was a hundred miles away.

At the end of July the St. Paul Fire Department came with busses to take us fishing. All the "walkers," most of the patients on crutches, and many of those in wheelchairs went. Our fishing hole was a channel just off nearby Lake Phalen. It was regularly stocked with fish, which were confined by nets on each end of the channel.

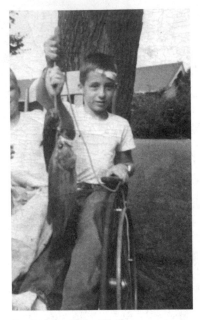

Fresh from Lake Phalen,
the winning bass

The firefighters brought fly rods along and showed us how to use them. The firefighters, patients, and staff all crowded along the shore on one side of the channel. After an hour, nobody had had a bite.

Just for the heck of it and to find an open space, I moved over and cast on the other side of the net, outside where the fish were stocked. As I reeled the first cast in, a fish bit the fly and hook about a foot from shore. I got excited and pulled so hard that the fish came out of the water, flew over my head, and landed behind me. A firefighter caught it in the grass with his hands and put it on a stringer. It was a beautiful five-pound bass.

Two fish were caught that day. Dennis caught the other. Mine was bigger. We took pictures of them and arranged to take them back to Gillette. I asked to have the kitchen prepare mine for my dinner that evening. When the hot cart came, I asked, "Where's my fish?" The nurses didn't know, they said, but they would check on it later.

The next day there still was no fish. I asked again, and Mrs. Beaver said she would check. When she did, the kitchen said they could not find my fish, but they would locate it by the next day.

The following day I was served a small piece of the worst smelling, stalest fish I had ever tasted. I knew from Grandpa Geislinger what fresh fish looked and tasted like. That was not my fish. Somebody stole my fish and ate it, I thought, and then went to the store to buy me the awful piece they cooked for me.

At home if you caught a fish, you got to help eat it. The incident reminded me: No matter how comfortable I was at Gillette sometimes, I was not at home.

The daily schedule at the hospital provided lots of other reminders.

The day always started early. The final duty of the night shift on the ward was to wake everyone up to brush teeth and wipe our faces and hands with a warm, damp rag. That had to be finished by six, so the nurse could tidy things up by seven when the day shift arrived.

The day shift barely had time to look around and get oriented when the breakfast hot cart rolled into the ward. It usually had a cereal, wilted toast (buttered in the kitchen), juice, or a fruit. Sometimes bacon, sausage, or scrambled eggs was included. Because it was prepared more than a half-hour before serving, it often seemed soggy and stale.

After breakfast, the morning meds were distributed. Then it was time for the "rescue squad," which consisted of someone pushing a large cart with cold stainless steel bedpans and urinals. All the bed-bound patients in the ward had to use these instead of the toilets in the restroom. This was a "do-your-job-on-demand" occasion for two reasons. First, the staff was inconvenienced when they had to deal with bedpans at other times, and second, you risked getting another enema if they thought you were getting constipated.

Next on the schedule were baths. Nearly everyone took one every few days, even the bed patients, who got bed baths.

After that, the beds were changed. If your linens were clean, they were changed after a few days. If they were soiled, they were changed right away.

After the noon lunch, it was naptime. During that very quiet time, the floor was mopped. Everyone who was not in school went to bed for an hour. If you did not sleep, you had to fake it. You could not even read.

The second shift arrived at three in the afternoon along with the "up" patients from school. The hot cart arrived at five with barely warm food that was not home cooked. After that, we played or watched TV until ten and lights out.

One of our favorite shows in 1951 was "The Lone Ranger." It was really exciting when Clayton Moore, the real Lone Ranger, came to visit us. He wore his mask, but you could tell who he was by his distinctive voice.

Afterwards, Don and I sat at Willie's bed admiring our Lone Ranger badges, which had small hidden compartments. Don had an arm that ended above the elbow due to a birth defect. Both of Willie's arms and legs were paralyzed from polio. My right leg had a cast on it. We realized that together we had three heads, three good arms, and three good legs. That was like one head, arm, and leg for each.

To make the time go faster, we started thinking of all the things we could and couldn't do in this condition. Horses had different strides, we knew, such as walking, trotting, and galloping. How many were there for people besides walking, skipping, and running?

To that list we added walking with crutches and one good leg. There were different ways to walk on crutches, but we knew the name of only the fastest, "the crossover." When you were doing the crossover, you could nearly catch someone with good legs. You could also fall and crack your casts.

The physical therapist showed us the safer "swing-to" and "two-point-alternate" methods, though she didn't call them that. We taught each other how to do the crossover.

Here's how it worked: If you had a good left leg, like I did, you leaned on the left crutch, tipped forward while bringing the left leg forward, stood on it, then did the same with the right crutch, the left leg, the left crutch, the left leg, etc. With practice, you looked like someone running gracefully with three legs, taking smooth, huge steps.

They sent me home after 38 days. Dad picked me up this time. I had a walking cast on my right leg, but no crutches. I didn't get any special treatment when I got home, though everyone was happy my leg was getting better.

Three days after I returned I discovered, during our usual Sunday noon dinner feast, that everyone now had a "favorite" piece of roasted chicken. I was last as the platter came around. Only a neck remained. I swallowed gamely and slid it onto my plate, proclaiming that it was my favorite.

It was partially true—our big homegrown roosters had huge meaty necks. Getting the piece that nobody else wanted also made me feel left out. I think Mother noticed. After that, anyway, she always left some breast meat attached to the neck when she cut it up for cooking.

I realized about the same time that no one at home ever asked about my stay at the hospital. Not a word. If I brought it up, my family changed the subject. It made me feel as if I had done something that embarrassed them. I guess maybe they thought of the hospital and polio as a bad thing, something that you shouldn't dwell on. It would have been nice to talk to someone about it, I think. We did not have a phone at the time, however, and I don't know who I would have called if we did.

Seventh grade started a few weeks later.

I got lucky in one regard. One of our teachers insisted that we had to have polished shoes. If they weren't shiny, we had go to the shoeshine stand in the back of the classroom and polish them. Since I had a cast on my right leg, I had only one shoe to polish.

Recess was a different story. We had to go down three flights of stairs just to get to the lunchroom. After lunch, the class ran up a flight of stairs and then a few blocks to the town ball field. I was always the last one to get there. By the time I arrived the various games were already organized and underway. I couldn't simply announce that I was on a certain team. Even if I could, I had a cast on my foot, so I couldn't contribute much. And I had to leave the playground early if I wanted to get back in time.

If I stayed back at the school, I was even more alone.

In March, my doctor realized the right anklebone block of the previous summer was not working. I was going to be pulled out of school again and admitted to Gillette Hospital for the fifth time.

3-4-52

Measurements from the anterior superior spine to the medial malleolus revels that the two legs appear to measure equal length today and we must be on the alert to remove the staples from his left knee should this leg get a little short. X-rays of the left knee shows six staples in the distal femoral epiphysis. The right foot still drops and a posterior bone block appears ineffective. This foot drop on the right should probably be corrected even if it means doing another bone block and one might also consider a tenodesis of the anterior tibial tendon right. He should report in a few weeks or else next Tuesday, for admission: Dr. Babb.

The following Monday, the day before I had to return to Gillette, Dad took our car to his brother Andrew's garage in Kimball for a tune-up and oil change. A car engine crankshaft had burned out on a trip back from Gillette a few years earlier. Now every trip to Gillette included this ritual.

On Tuesday, March 11, 1952, Mother, Dad and I hit the road once again. I already knew that I would likely have to stay for another operation. I felt helpless on that ride.

While we were waiting for the doctor, Dad told me a story about a boy who wanted something to play with and something to wear for Christmas. He could get only one thing.

"What was it," Dad asked.

After thinking awhile, I answered, "I don't know."

"Well, he got a pair of pants with a hole in the pocket. That's what he got," Dad explained.

The joke was so out of character for him. He had only ever told three stories that I could remember. He was trying to reduce the stress, I think, or raise my spirits. I thought it was funny, but I was so surprised I didn't know if I should laugh. Mother did not seem to think it was amusing.

It took three weeks before I had surgery this time, instead of the usual one week. Three weeks as a patient with no cast, no brace, and no crutches. Both legs were the same length. That meant that the old high sole on the right shoe was also gone. I looked nearly normal. Many patients and staff asked why I was there.

That was when it occurred to me for the first time that when I came to Gillette I usually walked into the hospital looking fairly normal and when I left, I usually had a cast and crutches.

I also noticed that in the hospital almost no one asked me about home.

Since I knew all the Ward 6 staff and many of the patients, I had the run of the place. For three weeks, I could play with crutches or wheelchairs. I could help others, show them how to go fast, or see who could go longer or faster on two wheels. I could join any patient at his bed to help build a model, listen to the radio, or play cards or chess.

As usual, I felt pretty lucky as I looked around. All the others looked to be worse off than I was, I thought. I would not wish to trade places with any of them.

I got a little scared when they again prepped both legs before surgery. Once again, no one explained to me in advance what they intended to do. The memories of the painful operation in January 1950 dominated my thoughts. That one was supposed to be the last one. Maybe this one would be. I decided that this time when I needed a hypo for pain, I would moan louder and ask sooner. Why wait until the pain made me cry?

4-1-52

DESCRIPTION OF OPERATION: The patient was placed in the prone position; and under general anesthesia, with the right side built up on sandbags, the left leg was raised from the table and bent at the knee so that from the knee to the foot the leg enjoyed a vertical position. A three-inch incision was made on the anterior aspect of the left tibia and was continued immediately through the deep fascia to the bone. A Luck saw was used to cut out a piece of cortical bone 2-1/2 inches in length and 1/2 inch thick in width...

Then the operator's attention was turned to the right foot. A three-inch incision was made through the old scar. ... The former bone block was found. It was weak, and there was a pseudarthrosis in the calcaneal insertion of the block. This was removed, and the hole in the calcaneus was enlarged. With the assistant holding the foot at right angles, the new piece of bone was pounded down into the calcaneus so that it was firmly anchored in the calcaneus and extended very nicely up behind the tibia. The bone was found to be so long that it interfered with the tendons which were to run over it, so about 1/2 inch was cut off and this, too, was pounded into the calcaneus to make the graft much firmer. Small bone fragments were then added; and, following this, the wound was closed in layers with #00 silk used in an interrupted suture for closure of the skin. ... A plaster cast was applied from below the knee to the toes of the right foot.

They took a piece of bone from my good left leg, below the knee, and put the piece in as a repeated bone block in the right ankle. A week after surgery, just when the pain was mostly gone, I developed an infection in my right foot, inside the cast. The outside of the cast was stained from

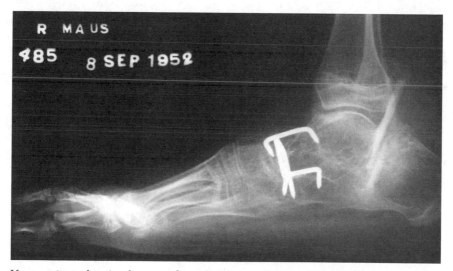

X-ray, 9-8-52, showing bone grafts and earlier staples to stabilize foot

the inside by the discharge. My leg smelled terrible. My temperature got as high as 104°.

The doctor ordered penicillin shots every three hours, day and night, for about four days. That hurt, especially since, in those days, needles were reused after being sterilized and sometimes got dull with repeated use. The nurse woke me for the shot if I was sleeping. Each arm and butt-cheek got two shots a day.

I was in Ward 1 for several weeks. All the patients there were bed patients. One of them screamed, moaned, and cried day and night for a week for a nurse to do something about the pain in his foot, but his leg had been amputated above the knee. Occasionally you could ask to have your bed rolled next to another for a game of chess, but most of the time was spent alone.

It took a while to eliminate the infection, but eventually they transferred me back to Ward 6. It was good to be back. A few cubicles had bed patients, but usually the patients were all over the ward. The lights went out at ten P.M. The older boys could watch the TV news for another half hour. Then everyone had to be in bed. It never got completely dark in the ward since the nurses' station had a light on all night.

A few times a year, lights-out marked the start of the fun rather than the end of the day. You knew when it was to happen. Everyone was looking over their shoulders, folding paper boxes that could be filled with water, and figuring out ways to get an extra stash of water. When the water bombs went flying in the dark, you had to be able to say to the nurse, "It wasn't me. See, I still have my water."

Water fights made two problems for the night nurse. First, there was lots of yelling and screaming. Second, she had to get dry gowns and bed sheets and change any beds that got wet. If only an edge or corner got doused, you got to wait until morning. When she got control at one end of the ward, the action frequently moved to the other. She was not happy.

Very often the event occasioned a visit from Miss Conklin, the hospital superintendent. You could hear her coming. She walked fast, determined, tall and straight. Earlier she had served in the military. You knew it when you saw her walk.

I think she thought she stopped the water wars with her arrival, but the truth was that we usually ran out of water and boxes about the time she arrived.

After every battle, for the next month or so, we were given only water glasses, not pitchers of water. While we waited for the nurses to let down their guard again, though, we had the fun of recreating the episode, deciding who threw where and hit whom.

The high school section of the *Gillette Echoes,* a newsletter put out by the hospital school, didn't cover water fights, but the May–June 1952 issue did note other entertainments, from swimming and archery meets to Boy Scout meetings.

The Ward 9 news noted a new "fashion" among the girls recovering there from operations, "collar casts." The Ward 8 news reported the death of a pet goldfish. One boy reviewed science fiction stories that he liked. Another offered a list of good books about airplanes.

I contributed a series of riddles, beginning with "Who was the fastest runner in the world?" The answer, on the next page, was "Adam, because he was the first in the human race." Another asked, "Why is a schoolroom like a car?" "Because the crank is usually in the front."

Visiting hours at the hospital were 1:30 to 3:30 every Saturday and Sunday. A patient could only have two visitors at a time, and children were not allowed.

The half hour before visitors arrived was the slowest of the week, and the two hours of visiting time were the fastest.

Mother and Dad came to visit every two weeks on Sunday as promised. I always cried when I saw them and cried again when they left. If my brother Phil and sisters Ruth, Helen, and Louise came along, they had to wait in the car. A patient could accept food or candy from a visitor only if there was enough to pass around the whole ward. Sometimes we cheated and they slipped me a small bar of candy or an apple.

I was ready to go home. In fact, I was getting homesick. I decided that the next time I saw him I would ask Dr. Babb if I could go home. When the time came, I was too intimidated by him and his entourage to ask. He did not explain anything to me and I did not ask.

I felt bad. Why hadn't I asked? I resolved to ask him the following week.

The next week was the same story. This time I felt even worse. Why couldn't I ask? Next week for sure, I would.

The third week, without my asking, Dr. Babb announced that I could go home.

Once again, I got home just about the time school let out for the summer. Within a month, though, I was back at Gillette, this time with an infected foot. I went to the operating room for "exploration" of the open wound three times before it healed properly.

9-16-52

His incision at long last is almost completely healed. He may start getting up now wearing the shoes he came in with and

start graded weightbearing in physiotherapy. He will require
just a dry protective dressing on his right ankle.
Measurements from the anterior superior spine to the sole of
the heel reveal that there is no gross difference in leg length.
He does not need any shoe build-up now. He does have a little
genu valgus of the left knee. I would like an AP and lateral x-
ray of the left knee for comparison with previous films. May be
up in the ward when ready. Dr. Babb.

They discharged me again on Wednesday, September 24. My eighth
grade class, I knew, was already three weeks into a new school year.

On the way home, between Buffalo and Maple Lake, Mother looked
over at me. "Why do you look so sad?" she inquired.

"I don't know," I answered. I was already missing my friends in Ward 6.

The following Monday I walked into school, climbed two flights of
stairs, and hopped into my classroom through the door in the rear. The
students were all in their seats. Nobody turned to look at me. The
teacher didn't even stop what she was doing. She simply pointed to the
empty desk in the middle, along the window row. I felt like I was invisible. I felt I existed only in Ward 6.

At recess, everyone scattered to the far corners of the playground,
playing chasing games. My only choice was to sit on the school steps
alone or hobble over toward some third or fourth graders who seemed
fascinated by my crutches.

It was 175 days since I had been at the school. Once again, I noticed
changes among my classmates, things that the students likely did not
notice and maybe not even the teachers.

One student was really different. For seven grades, he had been very smart, the smartest kid in the class. He always did his homework and dressed neatly. He was almost the teacher's pet. Now he skipped school, talked out of turn in class, and dressed sloppy.

I wondered what had happened. Could your life change from good to bad in just half a year? Could it go from bad to good that fast? From bad to even worse?

I also discovered when I returned that I did not have to do homework if I didn't want to.

At first, I had a good excuse. I had been absent the day before, the week before. After that, though, there wasn't any real reason. I just didn't feel like doing it. I guess the teachers didn't feel like making me do it, either. I managed to avoid doing homework for months and months.

There were more than 55,000 cases of polio in the United States that year, the most ever. The newspapers were full of scary articles about it. Many towns closed their theaters, swimming pools, and campgrounds. Parents cautioned their children not to play with anyone who had polio.

It had been 13 years since I had had polio, but my classmates seemed to think I was still contagious. They seemed to think I was different somehow. I wanted to think that it was just my foot that was different and that it was getting fixed. I wanted to think I was one of them or that someday I would be.

One day the teacher passed around a special "March of Dimes" can for coin donations from each student. She said that the money went for "people like Richard." I went home and asked Mother if I would ever get any of that money.

She simply said firmly, "No, Gillette is taking care of you, and it gets its money from the legislature, the taxpayers. The dimes collected in the March of Dimes go to others and is used to find what causes polio. Go to school and tell the teacher that, no, you did not get any of that money."

I was feeling very special—in a way that did not feel good.

I did a private experiment to see how long it would take someone to speak to me, about anything. How long would it be until someone initiated a conversation with me before school, before class, in class, at recess, or after school?

It was much worse than I anticipated. It took four days.

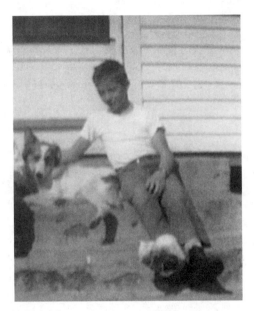

On the front steps in 1952 with my best
friend, Rex

CHAPTER 5

*O*n the farm, crippled animals were rare. There wasn't time to coddle them. Usually they died, or we shipped them to the South St. Paul stockyards.

Porky was an exception to that rule. Porky started life as the 13th little pig in the litter of a sow with only 12 feeding stations. Shortly after birth each infant porker claimed its own place to suckle. Porky was the odd man out, the runt. If something wasn't done and quickly, he was going to die.

Dad spotted the situation a few hours after the litter was born. He brought Porky into the house and placed him on an old rag in a cardboard box in the basement. A light bulb hanging above provided the warmth he needed. We fed him warm milk from a bottle with a nipple.

Since we were the first ones to nourish him, Porky imprinted on us. As he gained strength and grew, he depended on us for both food and attention.

We played with Porky just like he was a puppy. When we called "Here, Porky," he came running. At about 30 pounds, he was fun to roll over like a log in the grass. He used his snoot to roll us over on the lawn, too.

Before long, though, he got too big. We couldn't allow him to dig anymore in the flowers that Mother had planted around the house. It was time for Porky to join his siblings and half-siblings in the pen in the pig barn near the creek.

It could have been a disaster. Pigs can be vicious and he didn't have any experience dealing with them. But we didn't have to worry. In his very first pig-fight encounter, Porky came out the victor. Because of that, he became the boss of the whole pen.

When I walked into the pig barn later, all the other animals stampeded away from me in a cloud of dust and oinks toward two small exit doors at the rear. Not Porky. Instead he stuck his nose between the boards of the gate I was leaning on. He stayed as long as I scratched him.

I went back many times to study Porky. We had something in common, I thought. We were both different.

Did Porky know he was different? Did he realize how lucky he was to find a way to fit in when he returned to the pen? Did he ever miss playing with us on the lawn?

I also spent many afternoons petting and talking to Rex, our dog. I was not feeling useful or welcome. I did not feel needed. I didn't feel like I belonged.

In school, nobody invited me to do things with them. I simply tagged along. When my eighth grade classmates talked about who they liked, nobody ever asked me who I liked. They never teased me. It did not matter to them.

Was I even supposed to be here? I wondered. If I died, would anybody miss me?

If I were dead, I thought, the pain would disappear. I wouldn't feel so alone, so useless.

I could jump off the top of the silo. That might work.

No, I thought. That was too scary. Besides, I might only get hurt badly and end up in a hospital with a worse problem.

I could use our rifle.

What if the first shot didn't end it, though? Then what would I do? Even a rabbit sometimes took more than one .22 bullet before it died.

Why did I need to be here anyway? Why did everything have to hurt so much?

Suicide might be painful, I reasoned, but at least it was a pain that ended quickly.

Rex and I had many sessions on this subject. Sometimes we sat on the bridge, my feet dangling a few feet above the flowing creek. Other times we sat in the shade under a large box elder on the front lawn. We even took naps together. I told Rex how I would miss him.

Then I realized—he would miss me, too. Who else could spend so much time with him? Who else would take care of him the way I did? Who else would understand him as well as I did?

The answer was nobody.

Porky liked me, but Rex needed me. Rex would miss me. I had to stay around for Rex, I decided.

On two or three separate occasions late in the fall of 1952, pieces of bone, fragments from the graft, worked their way out of the rear of my right heel. The first time it happened, a red spot appeared, then an open sore, and then the end of the bone became visible. I pinched it between my fingers, wiggled it, and pulled it out. It looked like a broken piece of a toothpick. The skin eventually healed over.

A month later, another piece of bone came out.

In January of 1953, I found myself back in Gillette, showing them a bone fragment and getting my legs measured again. My good left leg was now almost an inch shorter than the one that had been affected by polio.

It was getting knock-kneed, too, because of the unequal effect of the staples they had inserted on each side of the left knee. The staples on the left, outer side, of the knee were preventing the bone from growing as planned, while the right, inside staples were bending, resulting in a noticeable bulge.

Dr. Babb decided the left staples should be removed. I was admitted to Gillette the same day and scheduled for surgery the following week.

1-6-53
The right foot and ankle are fine except that another little piece of bone has now come out posteriorly and there is no indications for treatment. His left knee is in more and more valgus and his left lower extremity is 2 cm. shorter than the right. I believe the staples should be removed from the distal femoral epiphysis at the left knee, removed from the lateral side only. Is to be readmitted and put on the surgery list for Tuesday, January 13. Dr. Babb.

1-13-53
OPERATION: Removal of staples, lateral side of left lower femoral epiphysis removal of staples and restapling, medial side of left lower femoral epiphysis.

I had been gone little more than three months this time. Many of my pals in Ward 6 were still there. When I arrived, they were hooting and laughing. After the nurses got me settled in, they told me what the commotion was about. They had just heard that the parrot on loan to us from Ward 8, the girl's equivalent to Ward 6, had gone back and caused a stir with several new words it had learned. Words that the girls were not supposed to hear. The girls had to cover its cage to shut it up. They tried putting it in a closet, first, but it swore even more.

The next day was Wednesday, the time for the usual bi-weekly, afternoon feature movie in the auditorium. The cartoons again reminded me of my early memory of being in the same auditorium eight years earlier, when I was five.

The staff rolled the beds back to the wards from the auditorium with the help of "walkers" like me (only one good leg needed). That was a new procedure, put in place because there had been an accident. A bed with a patient on each end of it had gotten out of control going down the school ramp and crashed into the wall at the bottom, near Ward 1. The helpers had been riding instead of guiding. The 8-year-old in the bed did not get hurt but the bed had to be replaced.

Dewey was new, too. He had never been in a hospital before. He sat on his bed with that "Oh, shit" look on his face. He didn't have the slightest idea what to expect. We did, though. So Ben, Rob, and I went over to talk to him and fill him in on hospital routines.

"What are you in for?" we asked.

"An operation next week on my leg," he responded.

In a few days, I was going to have my 10th operation. There were no surprises anymore and that was comforting. The anxiety about unknowns, I had learned, was always much worse than the events themselves.

We started telling Dewey what to expect. We described the blood cart experience, exaggerating the details a bit. When the nurse came that day with the tinkling cart, she tried to distract him so she could poke his finger with the knife blade hidden in the cork she carried. He kept jerking away, but finally she got her blood.

Since everything had happened as we described, we had credibility. We told him everything that would happen in the next week. We poured it on about the enema and the pain in the rear at the end. Ward 1 was full, so he also saw a few patients come to Ward 6 directly from surgery. He had to be wondering, as I had that first time, where his clothes and shoes were and if he should make a break for it.

I was an old hand at all this, by now. Before succumbing to the anesthetic in the operating room the next week, I asked if they could save the staples for me. They were going to remove the staples on the left side of the left knee and replace the staples on the right side.

"Sure," said the doctor. "We'll save them."

The second day back after surgery, I asked the ward nurse where the staples were. She said, after checking with the OR, that they must have lost them or forgotten them. I was disappointed—it would have been great to have a souvenir to show my friends.

A nurse gave me a lock box and a radio. The lock box contained a deck of cards, a set of jacks, a pencil and notebook. The other patients had received theirs during the Christmas holidays, a few weeks earlier. It did not matter that the keys were all the same. At least we had a private storage place within the bedside stand.

Now that I had a radio, I didn't have to yell across the ward when Teresa Brewer's "Ricochet" came on and ask someone to turn up the sound so I could hear it, too. Actually, they were already doing it without my asking, I realized. It was nice to have friends, especially ones who knew what my favorite songs were.

Aunt Hedwig and Uncle Henry Johnson and Uncle Johnny all came to visit the weekend after the operation. How all three got in the ward at the same time was a mystery. They did not have news from home, but it was good to see them.

The two weeks between my parents' visits was a long time. I got very sad when everybody around me had visitors and I did not. It helped if I pretended I had a book I needed to read or if I noticed that I wasn't the only one, that someone else didn't have visitors either.

Lying in a hospital bed day after day, there was lots of time to do things like try to roll over and learn to whistle three different ways.

There was time for weirder things, too. I discovered that if you stared at the clock on the wall long enough, it disappeared. You couldn't move your eyes to different parts of the clock when you were doing this. As much as your eyes wanted to move, you had to stare at the same spot.

Doing that could kill about 20 minutes.

Around this time I also mastered the art of looking at stereo picture pairs and seeing the 3-D image without the stereo-optican viewer.

In mid-February, after another 44 days at Gillette, I was sent home. Shortly after I returned, Rex got run over by the big tractor wheel.

Dad told me as soon as I got home from school that day. It had happened in the deep snow on the tobacco-shed road. Rex's back end was badly injured. His head and front legs appeared to be all right, and he looked comfortable, but he could not walk.

We took food and water to him in the hay barn and visited him often. His condition improved. Two weeks later, after milking, he barked from his bed in the hay barn, trying to help chase the cows from the cow barn below. The next day, after milking, he crawled from the hay barn, around the silo, and down the hill to the cow barn below. Rex had made it.

I felt even closer to him after this. We had even more in common. He had three good legs and one crippled leg and walked with a limp after the accident. When he ran fast, he would use the bad leg about every third step.

I thought I could also run fast.

When my teacher announced that he was going to hold basketball practice each day after school, I told Dad I wanted to play.

"Are you sure you can do it?" he asked.

"Sure," I responded. "My knee and foot are feeling fine. I can run, and my arms and hands are good."

I lasted about two days. Practice always began with running. Just because I could run on the tobacco-shed road didn't mean I could run on a basketball floor. The running with dribbling was just as bad. I had to quit. The only other choice was to continue demonstrating to myself and others that I just could not compete.

When I told Dad I was quitting, he did not act surprised. He just invited me to help him some more with the chores.

In the spring, our class took a bus to Cold Spring, 10 miles away, to visit the high school that we would attend in the fall. At the end of the day, back in Watkins, I got a ride home in the pickup with Dad.

"How was orientation today?" he asked.

"Okay," I responded. "But I don't think I am going to go to high school."

"Why not?"

"What else is there to learn?" I responded.

"Oh, you will like it."

In September, after a few weeks of class, I felt better about things. Just as in the hospital, my fears about the unknowns had turned out to be worse than the actual events.

I met some new classmates and learned some new names. I made acquaintances, but I did not know how to make or keep friends. I did not know why. I wished my bad leg were the result of something like a football injury or being run over by a bus. People would find that more intriguing than being crippled by polio.

Physical Science 9 was fun and interesting. I read the whole book in the first two weeks.

Sports were a problem. Everyone not directly involved in competing was expected to enjoy watching.

It was not fun, but I tagged along to watch the football games on Friday nights. After the game, there was a mad rush to the local café downtown. The place was full of students buying pop and candy, singing, talking, laughing, pushing, and jostling. I felt alone in the crowd. I wasn't with anyone. I was there only as an observer. Driving the 10 miles home, all I could think of was "How can I feel so lonely in such a packed setting, a place where I know so many people?" The next week was filled with more of the same.

Finally, by Homecoming I realized I needed to do something. If I wanted a date, I would just have to overcome my anxiety and ask someone. I did, and she accepted. We doubled with another couple.

Now that was real progress. Things were beginning to come together. Finally!

A few days later, on Tuesday, October 6, I went in for a routine checkup. The doctor admitted me to Gillette the same day and scheduled me for surgery the following week. I wouldn't get back home, back to school and those new beginnings, for another month and a half.

My left knee, the one on my "good" leg, was very tender on the right side. That side of the knee wasn't supposed to be growing, but it was. The left side should be growing, now that the staples there had been removed. But it wasn't. The lower part of the leg was 20 degrees out of alignment with the upper leg.

Dr. Babb removed the staples on the right side and replaced them with a bone graft that would guarantee no more growth there. That would prevent the knock-knee condition from getting worse, he hoped.

10-6-53
He has had no drainage from the right ankle for two months. Has had no pain. He has quite a marked genu valgus on the left, which measures 20 degrees today. He is acutely tender over the medial femoral condyle of the left knee where the staples appear to be backing out. This is the present problem for which he must be admitted at once. X-rays of the left knee, AP and L and right foot and ankle should be taken. Is to be scheduled for Tuesday, October 13, for removal of the staples and further epiphyseal arrest at the left knee. Dr. Babb.

10-13-53
OPERATION: Removal of previously inserted staples, medial epicondyle, left femur, and Phemister operation, medial epicondyle, left femur.

While recovering in the ward, I had plenty of time to observe the activities there. I tended to focus only on the things that moved. I had already studied the things that did not move for hours, days, and weeks.

The whole ward enjoyed watching one of the aides when she served cake. Every time she slid a fork under a piece of cake, she put her thumb on the top of it, in the frosting, to hold it in place. And after she served each piece, she licked off a thumb full of frosting. We just hoped that the frosting she touched stuck to her thumb.

A good book or a game of chess sped up the clock sometimes. One day a volunteer wandered through the ward, doing a different card trick at each bed. Sometimes he explained how to do the trick. He could fan a deck perfectly.

I returned home on Friday, November 13, 1953. I had missed six weeks of algebra. The girl who I had the earlier date with now had a new steady boyfriend. Not me. If only I had not had to go back to the hospital, I thought.

It took a while to catch up. Especially since I had decided again that I did not have to do any homework. How could I? I didn't know what they were doing in my classes or at least that's what I told the teachers. A few of them objected, but most allowed me to get away with it. I stretched it out for as long as I could.

I avoided studying, too, as a form of insurance. That way, if I failed a test, I could tell myself that it was because I hadn't read the lesson, not because I was stupid or something.

Sometimes I thought I was ready and failed the test anyway, possibly because of anxiety. That made the next test even more stressful, of course.

Things looked brighter in one area, though. My chorus teacher asked if anyone had had piano lessons. You had to know how to read musical notes to play the piano. If you wanted to learn an instrument, he said, you could join the band. He needed new members.

It sounded like a great idea. Except for sports, I did not feel disabled. I simply had a right foot (and now a left knee) problem. I could sit and play an instrument. I could be a part of something.

The band director sent me home with a trombone. Dad helped me assemble it. I blew anxiously, but only a swoosh came out. I took a deep breath and tried again—with the same result.

I looked at Dad, disappointed, and said, "It doesn't work. Maybe we should get a different one."

Dad smiled and said, "Here, let me try it." He did. This time it sounded like a trombone.

"How did you do that?" I asked.

He showed me how to tighten my lips and make them flutter while I blew into the trombone mouthpiece. It worked. Without a mouthpiece, the lip flutter sounded to my young ears like a fart. With one, it could produce a beautiful sound, the kind that Tommy Dorsey's trombone did when he played "Marie."

The director gave me some lessons. I practiced at home a few times. Bob Weber, sitting at my left in first chair, was a very patient and helpful tutor, too, especially with trombone positions. I was now in the band.

The next year, with the old seniors gone and the band getting more members, I was suddenly one of the more experienced "old-timers." It was a lot more fun being a sophomore than being a freshman.

The morning of February 16, 1954, was also fun. At 5:30 in the morning, Mother and I headed for a checkup at Gillette. It had snowed about five inches overnight. The snow on Highway 55 between Watkins and Kimball was undisturbed by any tracks, much less a plow.

Mother did not like driving in snow. I loved it, though, I had my driver's permit, and I had been driving around the farm for years. So she let me, at age 14, drive all the way to St. Paul and back. I don't remember anything about the checkup, but the drive—that was the highlight of the winter.

School had some good moments, too. In biology, my older sister, Ruth, helped me with a hydroponics project, soybeans in a bowl of water with a few drops of nutrients added. Dad and I checked them every day. If the leaves started to turn yellow, we simply added a few drops of nitrogen and the plants turned dark green again. I was very proud of that project.

Other topics got my attention in biology that year. Like "pecking order" in chickens, the ranking that occurs between animals when they live in close quarters. I had witnessed it in our hen house. If it was true with other animals, like wolves, it might also be true for humans.

That could explain a lot. I seemed to be at the bottom of the pecking order. The animals at the bottom often suffer and sometimes die.

I also learned in biology about the concept of a survival territory. Outside of its territory, for various reasons, an animal simply cannot survive. In nature, the teacher and text often emphasized, the weak and crippled were the early victims of predators.

That did not sound encouraging. In fact, it sounded downright depressing. I had to find a way to survive somehow, in spite of my legs.

At the end of sophomore year, during a routine outpatient visit to Gillette, Dr. Babb took one look at my left knee and decided he needed to do something about the previously noted 20-degree offset of the left lower leg. The good left leg, instead of being longer, was now a half inch shorter than my right leg. He ordered new x-rays of my legs. Two weeks later, he examined them and scheduled me for surgery. On July 12, 1955, I was admitted to Gillette for the ninth time.

6-28-55
X-RAY READING: An x-ray of the right knee is normal and the epiphysis appears to be almost closed, X-ray of the left knee

reveals the epiphysis to be closed, particularly the distal femoral epiphysis. There is a marked genu valgus present due apparently to overgrowth of the distal femoral epiphysis on the medial side. There is no deformity of the tibia. He can be scheduled for a supracondylar osteotomy of the left femur on Tuesday, July 19. I would anticipate doing the osteotomy from the lateral side and using a block of bone from the adjacent femur to keep the wedge open. Dr. Babb.

CHAPTER 6

*t*he summer of 1955 marked the beginning of mass polio vaccination efforts. Magazines, newspapers, the radio, and television were filled with stories about how the vaccine invented by Jonas E. Salk was going to eliminate poliomyelitis. By August more than four million would be inoculated against the disease that everyone dreaded.

I just wished it had happened 16 years earlier. Or that I had been born 16 years later. It was hard to think how much pain could have been prevented with a simple shot.

I spent most of the week before my 12th and—once again—"last" operation having fun.

There were many friends to welcome me when I returned to Ward 6 on July 12. That felt good. I discovered that I had moved up in the pecking order, too. I was 16, not a little kid. I was well known and liked, not a loner who could be picked on. I had had more surgeries than many of the other patients and more time-in-hospital. Instead of sitting alone worrying what was going to happen to me next, I was now in a position to support others and to tell them tales of past adventures on the ward.

There were more "up" patients than "bed" patients, so we spent a lot of time playing with the wheelchairs. The new shiny metal models had swivel wheels in front and big drive wheels in the back. They were much more stable and easier to control than the wooden ones with big wheels in front and coasters in the back, the ones I'd learned to use as a little kid.

We spent hours racing in the chairs, balancing on two wheels, and speeding down the laundry ramp outside Ward 6. You could coast almost the length of the ward with no hands. It wasn't without risk, of course. One boy injured his arm when his old-style wheelchair "ground looped," going into a horizontal spin that sent him crashing into a nearby bed.

When the weather was nice, we went through the double doors to an outside play area. It had swings and a slide. It also had a basketball hoop.

When my friends and I weren't shooting baskets, we were chasing the ball. That got pretty exciting sometimes, because the west side of Ward 6 was lined on the outside with six-foot-deep window wells. They channeled afternoon sunlight into the brace shop located below the ward. If the basketball accidentally fell into one of these wells, we raced to see who could retrieve it fastest. Sometimes a patient with a brace or cast "won," only to discover that he could not climb back out to the playground. When that happened, he knocked on a brace shop window. Someone inside would open it and help the stranded patient inside and upstairs, usually without the nurses becoming aware of the episode.

There were other diversions, too, including a visit from the Minneapolis Aquatennial Queen. She and her entourage entered the ward, smiled, waved, and left. I remember wondering how that was supposed to make us feel better.

I also spent part of the week getting reacquainted with the hospital.

Some things had changed during the 20 months I'd been away. For one thing, older patients were now permitted to smoke if they wanted to. Twice a day they could go to a room near the kitchen and have a cigarette or two. This was the hospital's answer to the problem of patients sneaking out back at night to smoke.

The smokers on Ward 6 were mostly "Red Wing boys," patients from the state reform school. They were rough, tough, and a little scary. They had a habit of engaging in disgusting spit-face fights. As more than one surprised and repulsed non-Red-Wing patient discovered, it was no fun to be on the receiving end of one of those.

The food hadn't changed while I was gone. That alone was enough to make me want to go home. It was bland, mushy, and warm when it should have been hot. The bread was usually hard and tasted stale. The meals were predictable.

At home, everything was fresh and varied. My mother knew how to cook. She made bread twice a week. Hot food was just that, and cold food was cold. We had all the delicious ice cream we wanted. I missed home cooking.

Gillette was like another world, I realized. It was what I imagined an orphanage must be like, or maybe a prison. It had its own rules, its own procedures. Time went slower there, especially when you were recovering. Connections with the outside gradually faded, then disappeared. "Getting out" and "going home" meant the same thing. You couldn't do either until a doctor ordered it.

Before I realized it, a week had passed and it was Tuesday, the day of my surgery.

This time I knew a little bit more about what they intended to do. They were going to sever the bone just above my left knee, straighten the leg out, and then let the bone re-grow. That would correct the 20 degree

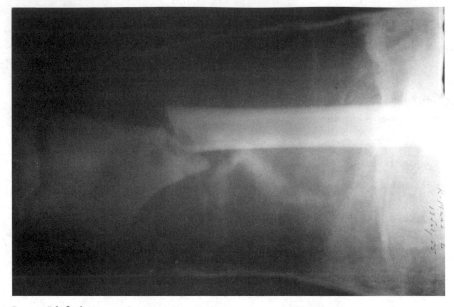

Leg as I left the operating room

knock-knee deviation caused by the earlier stapling. The knee joint would be crooked, but it shouldn't be a big problem.

Prep was routine. As usual, Mother and Dad weren't allowed to be there before I was wheeled into the operating room, but from previous experience I knew I would see them later in the day.

The transition from before surgery to after surgery was, as usual, instantaneous—and mind boggling. Before, I was comfortable. Afterwards, I was miserable—and just conscious enough to know that the operation was over. I spent the afternoon alternating between moaning, vomiting, sleeping, and waking.

Only one thing brightened an otherwise miserable day. When Mother asked how I felt, I told her, "With my fingers."

She then said to Dad, "He's okay."

She could not know it, but with my smart-alec answer I'd passed a test my friends and I had set up five days earlier. We'd been talking about the fog and confusion we experienced when coming out of anesthesia. We wondered if it were possible to program something different to say when people asked, as they always did, "How are you feeling?"

It took us a while to figure out exactly the right answer. I didn't want to say something obvious like "terrible." And only someone who was delusional would say he was "fine" when he was vomiting and passing out. I hoped I could remember to tell my friends that our experiment had worked.

There's nothing like pain to make time stand still. By dark, I was finally fully awake—and everyone else in the ward was asleep. I kept thinking, if only the pain was in the other leg or arm, I could handle it better. If it moved around my body, it would be easier. Having the same pain in the same place all the time was just so tiring.

I checked out my situation. I was in a body cast, I discovered. It stretched from the toes of my left foot, up my left leg, and around my torso to just under my armpits. Imagine using a cold, stainless steel bedpan in that condition. I knew I'd have to try. If I couldn't make it work, I'd get an enema to help. And when the skin under the cast started itching, and it always did, I'd just have to wait until it stopped by itself. There was no way to reach some of those areas.

It took five wretched days, but finally I began to feel better. That's when the doctor told me the leg needed more work. The x-rays they took before I left the operating room showed that the two bone pieces above the knee, created when they severed the femur, had not correctly aligned, end-to-end. It must have happened while they were putting on my cast. They intended to repair it the following week.

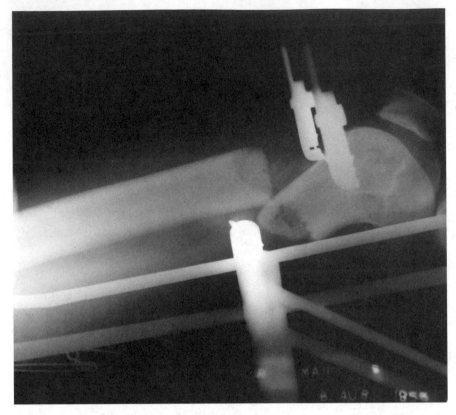

X-rays, left leg, 8-8-55: showing Kirschner wire and attached bracket, near the kneecap, upper right

Thursday came all too soon. After the usual preparation, I was back in surgery. The doctors removed the cast and then inserted a long thin pin horizontally through the bone just below the left knee.

This time when I came out of anesthesia, I found myself in a bed with my head slightly lower than my feet. Cables were attached to a bracket attached to the ends of the pin that protruded on either side of my leg. On the end of them, in a pulley framework at the end of the bed, were weights. The traction they produced was supposed to pull the bones apart slightly and allow the pieces to align correctly. The head of the bed was tilted downward to make sure that it was only the leg bones that moved and not my whole body.

It hurt a little, of course, and it was really uncomfortable. I couldn't roll over, and I felt sometimes like I was standing on my head. Worse yet, it didn't work. After several days, the x-rays they took showed that nothing was happening.

On August 4, they wheeled me into the cast room next to the operating room. This time they were going to give me a local anesthesia to block pain and enough general anesthesia to put me "almost" to sleep. That meant that for the first time I would be able to see what they were doing.

The doctor showed me a stiff, shiny wire with an end that looked like the tip of a 10-penny nail. He placed it in the chuck of an ordinary hand-operated carpenter's drill, placed it against my leg, and started cranking while another doctor leaned on the leg to brace it. Together they pushed the wire through the short piece of bone above my knee.

I had often wondered what it would be like to be awake during surgery. That day I found out. It was like wondering what it would be like to fall out of a tree or to be in a car during a crash. That is, nothing like the reality.

The doctors told me it shouldn't hurt much, but it did. It was also weird to see the pin pushing the skin outward, then poking through it from the inside to exit the leg. I had never seen anything like that before and I didn't want to again. By the time the procedure was finished, I knew I never wanted to be an orthopedic surgeon. There was no glory left in it for me.

The doctors rolled me back to the ward, where they attached another set of cables, pulleys, and weights to the new pin. They hoped that with the bones held in two places, they could pull them apart and manually poke and prod them into alignment. They came to my bed several times to try that. The manipulation hurt, but it did not work. I was scheduled for surgery August 9. It would be my fourth operation in three weeks.

Medical Record: 7-19-[55]
OPERATION: (1) Supracondylar osteotomy, left femur. F. S. Babb. M. D.
... The fascia lata was followed down to the inter-muscular septum. The muscle attachments in this region were then freed exposing the distal end of the femur. Multiple drill holes were then made across the femur in an oblique fashion.

... [I]n the process of the immobilization the fragments were felt to become unlocked. An x-ray taken at this time proved that the distal fragment had slipped posteriorly and proximally. In consequence, a wedge of the spica was removed and an attempt was made to manipulate the fragment into position. However, this proved unsuccessful. In consequence, the plaster was repaired and it was decided to put the patient in traction at a later date to achieve the desired position.

7-28-55
OPERATION: (2) Insertion of Steinman pin, the proximal end of the left tibia.
Under a general anesthetic, the left knee and calf were prepared and draped in the usual fashion. A Steinman pin was then inserted through the proximal third of the tibia. A paraplast dressing was applied and a traction bow fixed. The

patient was then placed in balance traction and returned to his room in good condition.

8-4-55
OPERATION: (3) Insertion of Kirschner wire, distal end of left femur.
Under local anesthesia and with x-ray control a Kirschner wire was inserted through the proximal end of the distal fragment of the left femur. It should be noted that a satisfactory insertion of the Kirschner wire could not be obtained due to the prior surgery and the position of the distal fragment.

8-9-55
OPERATION: (4) Manipulation of left knee under anesthetic.
Under general anesthetic an attempt was made to manipulate the distal fragment from its posterior position. This, however was not successful and, in consequence, the patient was returned to his room in traction.

The following Tuesday they put me to sleep and tried once again to pull and push the bones into alignment. When that "was not successful," I was scheduled for another operation. This time, they said, they would go in surgically, line up the bones, and, using four screws, put in a plate that would hold them in place.

I was a patient celebrity. Nobody else in Ward 6 had had that many trips to the operating room in such a short time.

By this time, I had been on pain medications and flat on my back (or tilted backwards) for nearly a month. What was supposed to have been one surgery was now going to be at least five. There was no guarantee, after all, that this one would be any more successful than the previous four. I had never heard of anyone dying in surgery at Gillette, but as they wheeled me into the operating room on August 16, 1955, I was beginning to seriously worry about it.

As I lay on the table, waiting for the surgeon to nod "ready" once more, I noticed a dark-haired nurse beside me. She was young, maybe a student. Her hand was on my shoulder. Her assignment was probably to keep me calm and occupied until it was time for my anesthesia.

It was kind of ironic, I thought. This was probably her first operation, but it was my 16th visit to the operating room. I welcomed the distraction anyway. I asked her about the big clock on the wall, the one with the numbers from 1 to 15. I already knew what it was, but it seemed like a good excuse to say something.

"That's for the tourniquet, so we can keep track of how long it's on," she explained.

I looked up at her again. Only her bright, beautiful eyes were visible above her surgical facemask. I asked her if she could it pull it down just for a moment. She glanced up at the doctor, then back to me and pulled it down past her chin. It was too bad, I said, that all the good-looking nurses had to work in the operating room where we'd never get to see their faces.

About that time, the doctor must have nodded to the anesthesiologist. I felt cool shooting into my arm. I woke up in Ward 6, vomiting, in pain, and encased in another cast.

8-16-55

OPERATION: (5) Open reduction and internal fixation, left femur, for correction of genu valgus.

... The fracture area was cleaned of all callous material and a reduction performed. After ascertaining good reduction a Moe-plate was put in place utilizing two wood screws at this lower and two regular screws in the upper end. The leg was held in the corrected position while fixation was accomplished. The stabilization was fairly good. A small amount of cancellous bone bank bone was then packed in the fracture site, bridging the open wedge on the lateral side. The fascia was then closed in the usual manner.

The day after the surgery I could remember having seen Mother and Dad, but just barely. It was getting hard to be sure of anything. The pain meds had started to cause hallucinations. In the most common one, parts of my body felt 10 times larger than normal. In another, I learned that my cousin had had an incredible accident. It was months before I realized that it had never happened, that I hadn't seen my cousin, that my "memory" was only a drug-induced dream. It had seemed so real. I began to understand how someone addicted to drugs could find it diffi-cult to separate reality from fantasy.

I was out of traction at last, but on my back still and in a full body cast. For more than a month, I hadn't been able to go to the auditorium movies. I couldn't see the ward TV, and I did not feel much like reading. I watched the clock a lot and stared at the ceiling. I was becoming des-perate to roll over. It became an obsession. I couldn't imagine anything better than being able to roll over and fall asleep on my stomach.

There were a few diversions. Hall, one of the other patients, hand painted a tie for me. The next time Mother and Dad came to visit they gave me $5 to pay him for it. It was amazing how what looked like a few streaks of paint up close could look, at arms length, like two ducks land-ing near some cattails in water. It was a treasure.

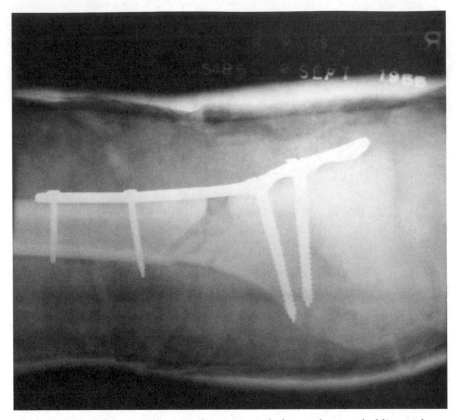

X-rays, left leg inside a cast, 9-2-55, showing metal plate and screws holding ends of bone in alignment

Then there was mail call. A half-hour beforehand, we started watching the nurses to see who was going to distribute the mail that day. I was getting a get-well card or two a week along with the usual letter each week from home. Some days, though, were perfect for the radio to be playing Earnest Tubbs' "No Letter Today."

On one memorable day the nurse's zigzag path around the ward included a stop at my bed. When I saw the name in the upper lefthand corner of the envelope she handed me, I blinked, too surprised and nervous to open it right away.

The previous week, feeling totally disconnected from the outside world, I had decided that I could not expect to get mail from classmates or have a girlfriend if I never wrote to anyone. I mentally went through the people in my class. It wasn't too hard to do—there were only 75 or 76 of us and I had gone to school with almost a third of them since grade school.

I decided to start with the one who seemed nicer than all the others, a girl from my sophomore English class. I wasn't sure if she knew that I liked her. My English teacher knew, though. When she reshuffled the seating chart, she kept us next to each other. She gave me a big smile when I looked at her afterwards, confirming that she knew and that I knew that she knew.

I opened the letter. It was short, but not very sweet. I read it at least 20 times, hoping to find something positive. I couldn't. It was nice hearing from me, she wrote, but she had another boyfriend. Everything was going great in school, she added, and I should hurry back. I didn't know what to think, what to do.

By lights-out, I was helplessly sad. I managed to roll myself over in the dark and I started crying uncontrollably. It felt good to be on my stomach for the first time in six weeks. At the same time, I was realizing that I had more than a foot or cast problem. I was bedridden. I had to use a bedpan. It felt like I was never going to get better, never going to get out of Gillette. How was I going to get a girlfriend at this rate? How was I going to get a life?

I cried myself to sleep, but woke up an hour later, needing to go to the bathroom. I had to call a nurse to help me roll onto my back so I could use a urinal.

In the morning, everybody and everything on the ward looked different. The whole world looked different. My best, much-considered effort to connect with someone on the outside had failed. I had no other ideas, no place to turn. If the hospital had staff to help with problems like this, I didn't know about them. I was alone and helpless. Compared to that the pain in my leg was nothing.

I wanted to scream as loudly as I could, "What is wrong with me?" To yell, "Somebody help me. Please!"

I cried myself to sleep every one of the next 11 nights, sobbing quietly into my pillow so nobody would hear.

I was going to have to solve this problem on my own, I finally decided. A few years earlier, talking with Rex, I had decided to stick around and see this thing through. I was going to make it, I vowed again. I was going to get past this. I was not going to spend my life this way.

By this time, I could roll over and back by myself. That was progress. I thought about how excited a mother feels when her baby rolls over the first time. I thought about how much a baby accomplishes in its first year. I could build on this. I *had* to build on this.

Within a couple of weeks I was getting around again on crutches. I started reading again. I buried myself in the *Amateur's Radio Handbook*. After a few weeks, I not only knew how a radio worked, I could make one if I had the parts.

I also searched out some positive things about 1939, the year of my birth, the year I got polio, and the year I was admitted to the isolation ward at Gillette. The movie *Gone with the Wind* had come out in 1939, I discovered, and so had the song "You are My Sunshine." It had been a bad year for me, but the year hadn't been a total disaster.

Finally, the doctor decided that I was ready to get out. It was mid-September. The school year had once again begun without me, thanks to the extra operations. I wouldn't be mobile enough to attend when I got back, but my leg was sufficiently healed to release me.

Dr. Babb noted on my chart that my left knee was now "nice and straight." He told my mother that I might need to have the plate removed at some point, but he didn't anticipate that I would need any further treatment since my left leg was now only one-fourth inch shorter than my right one, instead of nearly an inch. Holding the growth of the good left leg so the right could "catch up" had probably reduced my total height by about four inches, he said.

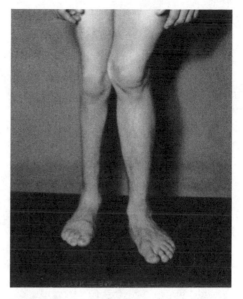

My legs in 1955, before surgery, showing effects of stapling on the growth of left leg

By the time I heard all this, my emotions were in neutral. I couldn't feel bad about it—or good about going home. I had always thought that when my legs got fixed, if they ever did, my worries would be over. I knew now that that wasn't true, and I still had no idea what to do to fix that problem.

9-12-55

DISCHARGED, Improved. He will not be able to attend school but I understand his assignments will be sent home to him. He is to return in 6 weeks and be admitted to have cast bivalved and checkup x-rays of the femur to include the knee, taken out of plaster. Dr. Babb.

9-13-55

The last x-ray shows the knock knee deformity to be well corrected and his knee is now nice and straight. Dr. Babb.

When I got out of the car, Rex took one look at me and started to whimper.

I said, "Hi, Rex."

He lowered his head, corkscrewed sideways in excitement, then lost his balance and somersaulted to the ground. Lying on his back, his legs up, he peed into the air and all over himself. I wouldn't have believed a dog could get so emotional unless I had seen it myself. Everyone could see how glad he was that I was home.

I was encased in a cast that stretched from my left toes to my armpit. I could get about on crutches, but not much more. Mother set up a bed for me in our large dining room, since I could not get to my bedroom above the kitchen. It was a challenge to use our tiny bathroom. It made a hospital bedpan look easy.

Mother told my youngest sister, Louise, to help me if I needed anything. She liked sitting around with me while Helen and Mother worked all weekend around the house.

On school days, it was very boring and quiet. Mother was busy in the house; Dad worked outside; Ruth was off to college; and Helen, Phil and Louise were in school most of the day.

I missed my friends in Ward 6. It was strange. In the hospital, I had wished I were home, and at home, I missed my hospital friends. Neither place seemed real to me. I felt like a disconnected observer in each place. Nobody at the hospital asked me about home. And at home, nobody ever talked about the hospital.

One afternoon I was showing off for Helen, goofing around the way we did sometimes at the hospital when nobody was looking. I was demonstrating how I could tip over like a falling tree and catch myself with my hands, stopping with my nose just an inch from the floor. The cast cracked behind the left knee. I went to bed. Mother contacted Gillette, and the next Tuesday I was admitted to Gillette for the 10th time.

Once again I was a bed patient in Ward 6. It was a week until I got a new cast, and then a few more days before it was fully dry. I passed the time playing chess and reading. A single game could burn up two hours in an instant. Only sleeping made time pass as quickly.

When I got back home, I asked Louise if she wanted me to teach her how to play chess. She said yes. We didn't have a chess set, so we created one with crayons and cardboard. I was excited. I had a chess partner, albeit a captive one.

I got more than I bargained for. Louise was determined to beat me. To the shock of both of us, it took her only a few weeks to win a game. Our games remained very enjoyable, but they got a lot more serious after that.

I couldn't say the same thing about my schoolwork. Helen brought home assignments every day, and I had the same old excuses for not doing them. How was I supposed to know what they were doing in school? In addition, what could the school do if I didn't do the work? Make me stay home? Ground me?

To my mind, homework was the least of my problems. I wasn't just missing physics and algebra II. I was missing band and goofing off with other students. Dad must have sensed that. By the last week in October, he suggested that maybe Helen could drive me to school each day, body cast and all.

"Can you do it?" he asked me.

"Sure, I can," I replied, forgetting about the stairs I'd have to climb, the doors and the bathrooms I'd have to navigate, and the books I'd have to carry while maneuvering on crutches through crowded hallways. I forgot that it was my "good" leg that was in the cast and that my weaker right leg would have to do most of the work.

I was desperate to avoid lying around the house for another six weeks, so desperate that I was willing to try anything. I wanted to show everyone that I was finally okay. That I was just like them.

Instead, I arrived in a cast in the back seat of a car being driven by my younger sister. That, together with the stairs, school desks that I could barely fit into, and arriving late with someone carrying my books, pretty much quashed any hopes I might have had of looking or feeling "normal."

People weren't seeing me, I knew, but my cast. Why couldn't my condition be more glamorous? Why couldn't I be someone who'd survived an airplane crash instead of someone who'd survived a virus?

Why couldn't I be a new student, for that matter? New students got to make fresh starts, got to make new friends and get involved in school activities. Instead, I felt like I'd been delivered to the wrong school, a place where I'd always be an outside observer. I was alone in the crowd and had no idea how to change that.

I had missed more than 10 weeks of school. I didn't care what I had missed in history or English, but I found it an interesting challenge to try to figure out what they had done in math and physics while I was gone.

I didn't have to go to physical education class. That was unfortunate, actually, since that was where friends bonded and weekend social plans were made. I was sent to the library for study hall instead. I was assigned to a table with five senior girls I knew. They thought it was fun having a junior boy with a cast at their table. After the librarian put a quick, firm stop to our socializing, I rediscovered how interesting libraries could be. I perused the shelves for anything that seemed interesting, especially astronomy books.

When it came time to have the cast removed, I only missed one day of school. My body was weak and stiff, but pounds lighter. My right foot was smaller than the left. My left leg was still slightly knock-kneed and a little shorter than the right. I would need to use crutches until I regained my strength, but the brace and thick sole of my childhood were gone.

11-8-55

The knee is clinically well healed. ... He should be seen again in about one month to six weeks for further x-rays before unprotected weight bearing is permitted. Discontinue shoe build-up.

I discovered quickly that fitting in wasn't just a matter of looking normal.

Now that the cast was off, I was going to be taking the bus to and from school. I was the last one to get on before it headed for Watkins. As a junior, I wasn't about to sit with the freshmen and girls in the front. Two books clutched between my right arm and its crutch, I hobbled down the crowded aisle toward the rear where my classmates sat.

Every seat had two occupants; most seats had three. The passengers had probably staked out those seats the first week of school and been sitting in them ever since. I was the only one standing. All eyes were on me. They were waiting, I knew, to see whom I would ask to move over.

Why couldn't I just get on the bus like everyone else, sit with my friends, and enjoy the ride home from school? Why did everything have to be some kind of contest? And why should some small, shy kid have to move over because I didn't have any friends on the bus? That wasn't fair.

I looked at the guy in front me, someone his friends called "Wild." We'd been classmates for 11 years. He knew me and I knew him. Our mothers knew each other. I asked him if I could sit with him.

"No," he quickly replied.

Everyone wondered what would happen next. It was my move.

In a split second, seemingly without thinking, I pulled my left hand from its crutch, formed it into a fist, and let him have it. As he sat there, stunned, blood started to stream from his nose.

I waited quietly while his friends offered handkerchiefs and shirts and helped him try to stop the bleeding. We were already past the S turn on the rutted gravel road and halfway to Watkins.

"Can I sit there now?" I asked.

Wild crowded over and I sat down beside him. Neither of us spoke a word for the rest of the ride, nor did anyone else in the back of the bus.

In school, things were getting more interesting. The band was increasing in size under the new director. I remained active in the camera and projector clubs and learned how to develop film and print pictures in the darkroom. If I came late to class, I could use the excuse that I had been in the darkroom.

Every Wednesday evening at about nine, I drove through Cold Spring to the dance hall in Richmond. I did not have any friends there, but I knew most of the patrons from Watkins and Cold Spring. Many of my classmates showed up. With live polka music and beer all around, there was plenty to observe. Each week you could expect a fight, usually outside and usually over a girl. The singing, laughing, dancing, and socializing continued right up until the one o'clock closing.

I usually stood near the bandstand. If there was nobody to talk to, I could always watch and listen up-close to the band.

One evening, a little before midnight, Frank M. walked up to excitedly tell me that Wild wanted to drag race with me on the road that went past the dance hall. That was surprising, since both of us had old cars. Was Wild trying to make up for the school bus episode of a few months earlier?

By that point in the evening, everyone else in the ballroom had had a few beers, including me. Assuring me that my '50 DeSoto could beat Wild's old Chevy, Frank begged me not to let Wild get by with his challenge. Then his friends joined in. It was intermission, they pointed out. Everyone would be watching this "drag race of the century."

At the door to the parking lot, I ran into Wild and more of Frank's friends. We got into our cars, started them up, and drove to the parking lot driveway. By then, quite a crowd of watchers had gathered.

When someone signaled the start, we headed west on the gravel road, flooring it.

As I ran up the RPM's in each gear of the stick-shift, I was not so much afraid that the engine or transmission would blow on the 6-year-old DeSoto, but that if something did fail, I wouldn't get the car again for a year. What I was doing was stupid, I knew, but I had to stand up to the challenge, didn't I? Nobody would have understood if I had just walked away.

The race was close. Neither of us could pull definitely ahead of the other before it ended.

I parked and walked into the ballroom. I found a hundred young, beer-drinking men and women looking at me and laughing. Nobody asked who had won. I moved around, watching, as the band played for the last hour of dancing, sensing that something was going on behind the scenes.

Finally, near closing, I asked a classmate what everyone was laughing about. Frank had set us up, he said. He told Wild that I wanted to race him and he told me that Wild wanted to race me. We were the butt of a big joke. The laughingstock. The fools.

And everyone knew it.

As I drove home alone, I wondered how I could have been so stupid. And why someone would want to do something like that to *me*.

The more I thought of it, the angrier I got. I would never even *think* of doing something like that to anyone else. Every time I saw Frank, the anger grew. While I was supposed to be paying attention to the teacher and acting interested in school, all I was thinking of was how mean Frank had been to me and how I could get back at him.

I could punch him in the face, but it would be obvious if I did so that I had started the fight. Besides he always had friends around, so that would not work.

I would have to surprise him. He would learn very quickly that there were consequences for picking on and making a fool of someone. And so would everyone else.

I could hardly look at anyone, I was so angry. Everyone had heard what Frank had done to me, I just knew it. I couldn't remember ever feeling worse, even when I was flat on my back in traction. I was supposed to be feeling better, now that I was out of the hospital, but I was feeling worse.

And why? Not for something *I* had done, but for something that had been done to me. Something *Frank* had done to me. If he were gone, I decided, I wouldn't have this problem any more.

There was only one way I could think of to make somebody gone.

That was with a gun. Shoot him. We had a single shot bolt-action rifle. It was old, but dependable. I had shot a lot of gophers and rabbits with it.

I would need to get it out of the house and onto the school bus. That wouldn't be easy. My parents didn't miss a thing. How could I get a rifle past them? I spent a few days obsessing about ways to accomplish that and about ways to get the gun into the school.

I thought about the consequences of what I was planning, too, but only now and then.

Someone would confiscate the gun, for sure, and I would probably spend the rest of my life in jail. Would that be so bad? I couldn't imagine anyone in prison being sadder or angrier than I was right then. Prison was bad, but it had to be better than the hospital. The food was probably the same, and there wouldn't be any surgeries or shots, any casts or wheelchairs. I was already alone. In prison, I would be able to read and think undisturbed all day if I wanted.

I spent days wondering if I really wanted to go through with it. Days trying to think of alternatives. There did not seem to be any. I couldn't talk with anyone about it, either. Mother or Dad wouldn't understand. Telling them how I'd been humiliated would only make things worse.

Then Robert, a friend from Gillette, came to visit. He lived near Alexandria. He had been passing by Watkins on Highway 55 and just decided to drop in. He drove into the farmyard and knocked on the door. When Mother answered, he asked, "Does Richard Maus live here?"

"Yes, he does. He's in the barn," she told him. She pointed to where I was milking cows. What a pleasant surprise it was to see him. We compared notes about our friends at the hospital and celebrated the fact that we were both finished there.

After he left, Dad stopped what he was doing, came over, and asked me, "Who was that?"

I explained that he was a friend from Gillette and that in the hospital I had drawn a map showing him where I lived. It was the first time since childhood, I think, that anyone had ever come to the farm to see me. I'm not sure what Mother and Dad thought about it, but it reminded me that there was a world outside of Watkins and high school and there were people who liked and cared about me.

It took a while but eventually I let go of what Frank had done and put my energies into better things.

I enjoyed the band. I could sit and play the trombone without my legs holding me back. Unfortunately, the new band director also wanted a marching band. As soon as the weather was nice and the spring concert was behind us, we started marching.

I didn't know how my legs would handle marching. Walking at my own pace and walking gently was no big problem. Marching to John Philip Sousa was a challenge, especially since the trombones marched in the front row, right behind the always-sharp majorettes. The band would set the pace, not me. I would not be able to stop to rub my knee or sit to rest my foot during a long parade. It didn't help that my shoes didn't fit quite right, either. We were supposed to wear white bucks for parades. We couldn't afford to buy two pairs of two sizes so Mother stuffed a wad of cloth into the front of the right shoe to keep my smaller right foot from slipping.

We marched in weekend parades all over Minnesota that summer. As my legs got stronger, it became more fun. It was certainly better than sitting home alone. I was in the band. I was starting to feel a part of something again.

Was that all it took? Feeling like I was part of things? I'm not sure. In any case, my senior year was fast and pretty bland. It seemed that nothing very interesting, exciting, or bad happened all year. I didn't become some kind of super student, but I did get more involved in classes. I'm not sure how my teachers felt about that, though. The yearbook that came out in the spring had the following quote under my picture: "There are two answers to every question, the teachers' and mine." Today I am very proud of that.

The year did have one unforgettable experience, though it didn't occur in school.

One nice fall afternoon at home, I slid open the big door to the hay barn, just enough to step through. I had done this a thousand times: Go in, pitch down some hay and straw for the cows below, then follow and distribute it.

This time, though, my eyes were drawn upwards, to the metal carrier mechanism hanging on the track that ran along and under the high peak of the barn roof. When we unloaded hay from a wagon, we positioned the carrier assembly so the rope and pulley could hook onto the bales on the wagon.

There was no hay to unload today, though, just some idle curiosity to be satisfied. I pulled the carrier into position. When the rope came down, I knew what I was going to do. I was going to see if I could climb the rope from the floor to the top at the peak of the barn roof.

There was nobody around to stop me, nobody to tell me it was crazy and I shouldn't do it. It should be safe, I thought. Every summer we filled the barn with hay and straw using this rope. The tracks up there were metal. The rope had never broken that I can remember. The same carrier, rope, pulley, and hook regularly lifted 10 bales at a time. I weighed much less than that. The rope and pulley would remain motionless, and if I fell the thin layer of straw on the floor might cushion me a little.

I studied my leather gloves, then the carrier above. I had climbed short ropes before, but getting to the top was only half of the task. What if I got exhausted at the top? It was a long way down. Who would know if something happened?

I removed the leather gloves. My hands were calloused. I wanted to feel the rope, especially if it slipped, so I could tighten my grip.

I glanced toward the door and outside, taking what might be my last look at sunlight. It felt good. I reached up, grabbed hold, and pulled. I was off the floor now; there was no returning. The faster I went, the better my chances would be.

I did not even try to use my legs. If I were to accomplish anything, it wouldn't be because of them. They dangled, not even touching the rope, as my arms pulled me upward, hand over hand. I reached the top of the rope at the metal carrier, the halfway point, and started down. It should be no harder, I thought, just more hand over hand, but down.

At the bottom, I didn't let go of the rope. The trip had been easier than expected. So was my decision to keep going. Up the rope I went again, hand over hand.

I had begun this effort just to see if I could do it. Now I was going as if a clock were on me or someone were chasing me.

At the top, holding the rope with only my left hand, I stretched out with my right, reaching up and around the carrier to touch the track. I wasn't sure why; I only knew I had to touch the track. It was important, like touching the bag when rounding third. I also knew I shouldn't look down; in the cartoons, when a character ran off a cliff, he didn't fall until after he looked down.

In a few moments, I was standing where I started. The feeling was indescribable, like hitting a grand slam or intercepting a pass and running 95 yards for a touchdown to win the game, bringing the crowd to its feet and driving it wild. Did you see that, did you see what Richard just did?

As I released my grip on the rope and glanced around, it hit me. I was alone. No one else had witnessed this amazing feat. I could not even think of anyone I wanted to tell about it. If I told Dad, he'd probably say, "If you've got that much strength and energy, I've got this other job for you." Anyone else would likely respond, "So?"

Remembering why I had come to the barn, I got some hay down for the cows, grinning all the while. Nobody else knew what I'd done, but the memory was vivid in my mind, ready to be replayed, in slow motion and stop action, whenever I wanted it. It still is.

We continued marching in the band, five of us, even after we graduated. Instead of riding the band bus, we drove our cars. A series of community festival parades culminated in the longest and best of them all, the 1957 Minneapolis Aquatennial Parade. We won first place.

I had been accepted at St. John's University, located in Collegeville, Minnesota, just a few miles beyond Cold Spring. Dad had attended high school there and always assumed that I would go there, too. Surprisingly, I did not think about college all summer. At least I tried not to. A lot of my high school classmates would be there, but so would hundreds of guys I'd never met.

What would it be like to be one of a thousand or more? Would I fit in? I hoped so, but I had to wonder: Why should college be any different from high school and the years before it?

i arrived at St. John's in the fall of 1957 with a lamp, a portable type-writer, a pair of shoes, and some clothes. I was assigned a double in Benet Hall, the dorm nearest to the quadrangle, the main classroom and dining hall building at the center of the old campus. Outside my window, workers were constructing the bell banner designed by Marcel Breuer for the new abbey church.

My room was on the ground floor, so moving in was easy. Fitting in was the challenge.

The first night in the room was very similar to being in a room at the hospital. It was not completely dark, and I could hear sounds from other rooms. Instead of worrying about an operation, though, my mind was filled with thoughts like: "Will I be able to make friends?" "Can I pass the courses?" "Am I ready for this?" I had no one to talk with about what to expect.

My roommate arrived the next day. He'd grown up more than 150 miles away, but he seemed to be right at home. He was friendly, confident, talkative, and ready to get on with college life. I was less than 30 miles from home, but I was shy, scared, anxious, and utterly lacking in confidence.

It took a while, but I finally met some of my new classmates, just by being in the room, going to lunch, and getting in and out of nearby rooms. I noticed one problem right away. My roommate could spend an hour with the six classmates next door and remember all their names; I had a hard time remembering even one.

The guys on the floor were fairly friendly. A few even asked me to join them outside for touch football or soccer on a couple of fine fall afternoons. Other students from Watkins, Cold Spring, and Richmond knew that I had had polio, but nobody else did. I had a slight limp, but it must not have been very noticeable. Still, I was afraid that the physical activity would dramatize all the things that I couldn't do. So I told them I needed to study. Eventually they stopped asking.

I *did* need to study. The problem was that I hadn't learned how to study any more than I had learned how to play football or soccer. In the end, I spent more time worrying about studying than actually doing any. When others wanted to study, I found someone who wanted to goof off. When others wanted to have fun, I said I was going to study—but didn't. When I saw others walking across campus, I thought, "If they are not studying, why should I?"

On the few occasions that I seriously tried to study, I ended up staring at my open book for hours, distracted by questions like "Why am I here?" "How can I feel so alone in this dorm full of men?" "What do I want to do? What do I want to be?" "What will happen if I don't make it?"

It was very similar, I realized, to the way I had whiled away the hours when I was at Gillette. My mind, maybe out of habit, was acting the same as it had when I was stuck in a hospital bed, thinking of everything and nothing at the same time.

Sometimes, hoping to break out of the funk I was in, I'd take a shower, read another James Bond novel, or go to the bookstore for a magazine or some tobacco. All too often I discovered when the lights went out at 11 that I had not studied a single minute all day. The anxiety that this induced made it very hard to sleep.

Since I rarely got a good night's sleep, I usually awoke feeling tired. The naps I took, sometimes two or three a day, became counterproductive; they made sleeping at night even harder.

I was able to keep up in the courses where I liked the instructor or the subject, like physics. Simply by going to class and paying close attention, I could get A's and B's on the tests there. Other classes like English or history I sometimes skipped altogether or I tuned out the instructor while I wrestled with my own thoughts. In one class an instructor had to ask me to stop talking to another student out of turn. I was embarrassed, but I thought, I'm required to take this class, but you can't compel me to be interested in it.

If I liked the class, it was easy. If I did not like it, the class was a disaster.

I was doing well in physics. It had been my favorite class in high school, and I thought I might major in it. The lectures and demonstrations at St. John's were interesting, and the tests were mostly multiple-choice. The first semester I got a B with only about two hours of studying.

Trigonometry was a slightly different story. I went to class each day knowing that I had to pass trig if I wanted to major in physics. The subject was almost totally new to me; we had had only about a two-week introduction to it in high school. Still, I didn't do a single minute of study outside of class. As the first test approached, about a month into the semester, I decided that I should at least do some review. I studied for about an hour, and to my surprise I got a 93, an A.

I tried the same strategy for the second test. It didn't work as well this time. In fact, I failed the exam. Now I was behind. I continued to go to class, continued to pretend everything was all right, but I decided that it would so hard to catch up that I didn't even try.

I wasn't doing much better outside of class. Looking over the options for extracurricular activity, I had decided that the rifle club looked interesting. I shot rifles and shotguns at home, after all. It took only two target practice meetings to discover that marksmanship wasn't as easy as it sounded. Legs were just as important as arms in most of the shooting positions. I could not imagine getting good enough to prove to myself and to others that I could do something well. After the two meetings, I quit.

For the rest of the year, I hung around the students I knew from high school, but I had no luck making new friends. I could talk with others, I discovered, but I had no knack for dorm room banter. There were so many things I didn't understand, and I was too shy and insecure to ask questions. Take my confusion about the Dean's List, for instance. Sometime during freshman year, I overheard one person laughing at another for being on the "Dean's List." I erroneously concluded it was a list of students who were in academic trouble and decided I didn't want to be on it. Since it was really a list of people who had done extremely well academically, there was never any danger of that, unfortunately.

After a year and a half of fitful and sporadic progress, I began to spend a lot of time on my own, thinking. I even skipped classes to think.

My classmates all seemed to know what they wanted to do. I did not have a clue about what I wanted for a career. In less than three years, they would graduate. I'd still be sitting here, wondering what I was doing. What a depressing thought.

I went to the quietest, most isolated part of the abbey library to do some serious thinking, a place where students and even monks rarely visited. I ate just one meal a day most days and slept most of the rest of the time.

Instead of clarifying things, this only increased my anxiety. I thought now and then of quitting, then I shoved the idea away. What would my parents think if I quit? How could I make a living? I had never had a paying job. Could I "make it" without a college education?

Why was I having this problem, anyway? Was there anyone I could blame? Could I salvage anything if I changed my major?

I could quit, a little voice whispered.

Nobody likes a quitter, said another.

Wasn't quitting like shouting "I am a failure" in the same way that walking with crutches shouted "I am a cripple"? I didn't like to take showers where others could see the scars on my legs or the fact that they were different sizes. Was I prepared to have people stare at me for yet another reason?

It didn't make any sense to keep doing something that was going badly. If you accidentally stuck your hand into a flame, you wouldn't keep holding it there, would you? You wouldn't run across a road if a car were speeding down it? It was stupid, wasn't it, to keep driving if you were running out of gas or to keep running if you could barely breathe?

If I quit, though, how could I tell my classmates? How could I tell my parents?

Finally, a little way into the second semester of my sophomore year, I decided that I simply had to leave college. There was no way to salvage things that I could see. It was only going to get worse. I did not know what I'd do next, but this wasn't working. I had to quit.

It was amazing how much better I felt once I made my decision. I felt about a hundred pounds lighter. I could read a whole article in a magazine in the library without getting distracted. I wasn't anxious any more. In fact, I felt good. I felt relaxed. That told me I had made the right decision.

I needed to figure out how and when to announce my decision to Mother and Dad. They might not be happy to see me at home again. Still, I'd be available to help on the farm, at least for a while. I couldn't imagine milking cows for the rest of my life.

It would be better if I could tell them that I had found a job. But what kind of job?

I decided to hitch a ride to St. Cloud and apply for a road construction job. I could drive a tractor or truck. I heard the work also paid well.

I was oblivious to the fact that the economy was at its lowest point in decades. It was winter, too, a time when construction jobs were usually scarce. On top of that, I had no real experience and no connections.

When I finally found a place where I could apply, I was courteously told, "You need to talk to the road foreman."

I didn't know what a road foreman was or where I might find him, for that matter. Even if I had, I wouldn't have had a way to get to him. Having a car wasn't necessary for attending college, but it was going to be crucial for getting a job and getting myself to and from work, I realized. Discouraged, I hitched back to campus.

The following Sunday I hitchhiked home, arriving at about noon, when I knew my parents would be there. Mother stopped, surprised, when I walked through the always-unlocked front door.

"What are you doing here today?"

"I'm quitting college," I responded, anxious to get things out into the open.

She could tell this was serious. After a pause, she said, "Well, Dad's still outside. You better go tell him."

It was bad enough saying it once. Now I would have to say it again. On the other hand, Mother hadn't objected or tried to talk me out of my decision. It was almost as if she had expected it. That didn't make it easier to face Dad, though.

I went outside and met him coming in from the barn.

"What are you doing here?" he asked.

"Hi. I'm quitting college," I answered. "I don't like it, and it's not going well."

"What will you do, then?" he asked.

I paused and then blurted, "Well, I could maybe farm."

At those words, he lost control and started crying. We just stood there for a while. I had never seen him cry before. This was going so much worse than I had imagined.

"Maybe I could go back to college in a year or so," I offered when he stopped crying. We pulled ourselves together and walked quietly to the house.

My parents agreed that it was a waste to spend money on something that was not working. Dad said that I was welcome at home. There was a lot of farm work, and he could use my help. I slept better that night than I had in months.

They called St. John's the next day, I think, to find out what the procedures were for dropping out maybe or to see if college officials thought I was making the right decision. In any case, on Tuesday, when I returned to campus to get my stuff from the dorm, the college and my classmates already knew I was leaving.

Before I left, I had to go to the Registrar's Office and take an MMPI (Minnesota Multiphasic Personality Inventory) test. Developed at the University of Minnesota in the late 1930s, it was designed to help detect psychological problems. I don't think I knew that then, and I never learned what my results meant. I just knew when I was through with it that I felt like some kind of failure.

Before I got my belongings and left, I dropped by one of the rooms down the hall. The first thing I noticed there was a chessboard with an incomplete game on it. When one of the guys said his opponent had had to leave before they could finish their game, I offered to take his place. I'll never forget the look of astonishment on his face when, within two moves, I captured his queen and began chasing him all over the board. (His opponent, it turned out, had actually forfeited the game, seeing no way to avoid defeat.)

The incident was a rare bright spot in an otherwise lousy day. I knew somehow that I would remember it a long time.

I was also sure that nobody would miss or remember me after I left St. John's. I had never felt I was a part of the place.

By spring, it was clear that I needed to get a job off the farm. I was nearly 20 years old, I had no money, and I owned nothing beyond a few items of clothing.

Dad alerted me to an opening in the cheese plant in town. In all likelihood, he had talked to the plant manager about it for he knew exactly what it entailed: waxing, weighing, and boxing 60-pound cheddars of cheese.

It was great having a responsible, paying job and money in my pocket. It was not so great paying room and board at home.

The job ended in mid-summer when the plant stopped making that kind of cheese. I was unemployed again. After a few days, I mentioned the idea of working road construction. It turned out that Dad had a pal from childhood who was now a road construction foreman. In fact, he was foreman for the St. Cloud company that I had visited six months earlier! Stranger yet, we ran into him in Watkins the very next Sunday, at a church dinner.

Dad had known the man since he was 12 to 15 years old; my grandparents had provided a home for him when his family fell on hard times. They reminisced a while, and then Dad asked if he had any openings.

If there wasn't an opening to begin with, he made one for me on the crew working on Highway 23 near Clara City. There was a problem, though. It was customary to do manual labor before graduating to driving. Knowing of my polio situation, he had assigned me to drive a tractor pulling a packer. Some of the other workers resented that.

At the end of the first day on the job, I felt like I had the world by the tail. The work was doable and the pay was great. By the next day, I was bored. Back and forth I drove, a half mile each way, packing the sand.

I thought I might get a break on the third day when it started to rain, but they told me that was the best time to be out there. The sand packed better when it was wet. I didn't mind the rain so much, but I didn't like the thunder and lightning, especially after a bolt flashed about 30 feet from my face. It was bright, loud, and very scary.

Then, for about five days, they did not need packing. I had to check in every day, though, just in case. That was followed by five straight days of good packing.

Packing wet sand was great, but wet dust turned into mud and packing that was just a pain. Unless you poked it out of the wheels right away, the stuff dried hard as a rock. The pain of keeping the packer's 16 wheels in good condition, together with the monotony of driving the same stretch of road over and over, got me thinking that maybe college wasn't so bad after all. At least there I could choose what I wanted to do. I could read. I could explore things that I found interesting.

After a year or two at St. John's some "Johnnies" transferred to the University of Minnesota in Minneapolis. Maybe that's what I should do, I thought. Give myself a fresh start. I had a better idea of what college was all about now and what courses I liked. That meant that I'd do a better job.

I applied to the U and was accepted. Classes started at the end of September.

i was going to pay my own way this time. My parents, who had two other children in college in the fall of 1959, hadn't offered me financial assistance, and I hadn't asked for it. I wanted to prove myself, for one thing. For another, in the event that things didn't work out, I didn't want to be guilty of wasting their money again.

After paying first-quarter tuition (just under $300) and rent ($35 a month), the nest egg saved from my paychecks was down to about $300. I was going to have to be very careful, I knew. This wouldn't last more than a few months.

The University of Minnesota had one of the largest enrollments in the country. It was also physically big. Walking across the campus was a real chore. Luckily, I had found a second-floor room in one of the oldest and closest rooming houses in the area. It was located on Walnut Street, just off Washington Avenue, across the street from Memorial Stadium, home of Gopher football.

Unfortunately, there was no off-street parking for my car, a '55 Plymouth bought used with more than 110,000 miles on it. Parking at the curb was limited to two hours. I tried to be diligent about moving it—or at least about driving far enough forward or back that the chalk mark the traffic cops made on the tires got shifted some. I ended up with a lot of tickets anyway.

In a surprisingly short time, I made a couple of friends at the rooming house, Jack and Jim, twin brothers with a large room on the same floor as mine. One Saturday they invited me to come with them to the football game.

It was a nice day. The game was less than a block away. I had a student season ticket so it wouldn't cost me anything. Before I knew it, though, I told them I needed to stay home and study.

I spent the afternoon with my book open to the same two pages. As I listened to the game on the radio and heard the cheers and the groans of the crowd across the street, I tried to figure out what was going on. Why was I doing the same stupid things I'd done a year or two earlier? I was supposed to be making a fresh start.

My funds continued to dwindle. It wasn't fair, I thought, my frustration fanned by the reading that I was doing in one of my classes about communism and capitalism. Why did I have to worry all the time about money? After all, at home and in the hospital food, clothing, and shelter had been provided.

I contemplated doing something drastic, like throwing a brick through a jewelry store window and standing there and waiting for the cops. I'd get food and a place to sleep in jail, wouldn't I?

Deciding that there had to be a better answer to my money problems than getting myself arrested, I started to look for a part-time job. I checked every bulletin board on campus, every issue of the *Minnesota Daily* newspaper, every flyer that was handed out, looking for a suitable job near campus. Finally, I spotted an ad for part-time student workers for the food service at the University Hospitals, located just a few blocks away.

I was familiar with hospitals and comfortable in them. There were openings for late afternoon and weekends, times when I could work. I applied, interviewed, and got the job, which consisted of setting up trays, serving food, and washing dishes.

I wouldn't get paid until a month after I started, naturally. I would run out of money before that; tuition for the next quarter was due shortly.

Jim and Jack loaned me $100, but I was still short. I walked into the nearby bank and—instead of robbing it—asked for a loan of $150. A bank official explained that the smallest loan they gave was $300 for six months. I took one out. I should be able to handle repayment now that I had the hospital job.

Fretting about money and getting a job took its toll on my class work.

In math, we were studying a topic that was new to me: permutations, combinations, and probability. I understood what the teacher covered in class each day, but I had not done a single one of the homework practice problems since we began the unit three weeks earlier. I needed to catch up—and in a hurry. There was going to be a test the next day.

I got the afternoon off at the hospital. At two o'clock, I cracked my math book open, ready to spend a few hours doing problems. After three hours, I had practiced and mastered only two sections—out of about 12—in the chapter.

Over dinner, I tried to decide if I should wing it and go to the test unprepared or stay up all night studying. I decided to study. However long it took, however late it got, I was going to do all the odd-numbered problems in the unit, the ones that had answers in the back of the book. Making sure that I had an adequate supply of popcorn, beer, cigarettes, and coffee, I dug in.

I went through the material, problem after problem, example after example, and section after section, checking my answers in the back. If I found that I'd given a wrong answer, I went back to the question and hammered away at it until I understood where I'd made my mistake.

By midnight, I was half through the chapter—and about half through the beer and popcorn. I was feeling wide awake, but at that rate it was going to take all night to finish. Before I knew it, it was getting light outside and I was nearly to the end of the chapter. The beer and popcorn were gone. The test was three hours away.

I finished the chapter, did the chapter test, and checked it. It verified that I had learned how to do the problems—and with an hour to spare. I grabbed breakfast and more coffee and headed across campus to Folwell Hall. I felt more awake and alert than if I had had 10 hours of sleep.

I got the test, went to work on it, and found no surprises. Everything was fresh in my mind. The problems were just like the ones I had practiced. In 45 minutes, I finished them all, neatly showing each step of each problem. I got up and turned in the test. It felt very strange to be leaving early. I had seen students get up and turn tests in early before, but I'd thought that if I ever did that it would be because I knew absolutely nothing about the material. For the first time, I realized that some students might leave early because they knew the material well.

Two days later, I got the test back. 100 percent. All correct. Perfect.

I'd finally discovered the secret to succeeding at college: Don't do anything for three weeks and then stay up all night and study. I tried this technique in another class. This time, though, I fell asleep during the test. Bad theory.

I did not get home until Thanksgiving or Christmas. When I arrived, Dad asked, "Why don't you write or call us sometime?"

"There wasn't anything important enough to write home about," I responded.

Was that true? After all, I had met a few interesting students, both male and female. On the other hand, I hadn't made any really good friends.

I did not want to be dependent on or obligated to anyone, I told myself. I was just naturally a loner. In truth, I did not know how make good friends any more than I knew how to study effectively.

I got an A in math that quarter and passed the rest of my classes easily, but I'd fallen back into the pattern of not studying in classes I did not like. I forgot to go to class sometimes and skipped tests in required classes several times because I was "too tired."

That cost me in more ways than one.

Thanks to the A in math the previous quarter, I had gotten into an honors calculus section. One day before class, the professor asked if I was interested in a scholarship. If so, he might be able to arrange for one.

"Sure," I said. It would be wonderful to not have to worry so much about money.

I think he checked my transcript and discovered that I had cut a few classes. In any case, when he got back to me a few days later, he said, "Sorry. No scholarships are available."

I attended the first summer session at the university, mostly in order to keep my student work job in the food service. It was interesting being on the other side of hospital care. I got to experience firsthand, for instance, why it was difficult to provide patients with food that was tasty and the right temperature. The food was hot when the cooks put it into big containers on the "hot carts," but by the time we pushed the carts to the various floors and ladled it onto plates for the nurses to take in to the patients it had frequently turned into lukewarm mush.

That didn't concern me as much as it had when I was a child. In fact, by this time I was doing most of my eating at the hospital. Putting left-over pork chops, mashed potatoes, and bread to personal use wasn't exactly permitted, but if we kept out of sight of the dieticians we could get away with it.

I got a leave from the food service during the second summer session and got a job as a bellhop at the Minnesota Hotel, a rundown place on Washington Avenue. Few of the guests needed help with their baggage, but the hotel was old enough that the elevators needed operators. After a week, I learned the position was a temporary one; it would end when the regular bellhop came back from a two-week vacation.

I contacted a guy that I'd worked with at the cheese plant in Watkins. He'd told me about a ranch job that he'd had in Montana the year before. It was a seasonal harvest job that involved driving a combine, herding cattle on horseback, fixing fences, and hauling straw bales. I sent an inquiry to the address he gave me. In a few days I received an invita-tion to come out right away and to bring my brother Phil, who was also interested. The harvest was going to start soon. We'd be part of a crew of two dozen guys.

We drove 17 hours straight to get to the ranch, which was located south of Chester in north-central Montana. When we arrived, we were shown to bunks in a dilapidated five-stall garage that had a decent roof but was open to the wind and weather across its front. Prairie stretched around us in all directions, interrupted by the Rockies to the west and the Sweet Grass Hills to the north along the Canadian border.

We cleaned grain bins for a day or two, then we were out in the fields harvesting wheat. Driving a combine in a row of 10 huge machines was thrilling—until you had to drive two-and-a-half miles with a slow breeze on your back. By day's end, wheat chaff and dust covered your whole body—and coated the inside of your lungs. It was miserable.

When it rained hard enough to prevent us from combining, we were assigned other tasks, like fixing fence or picking rocks. We also hauled bales. It was a four-man operation. Running along one side of a slowly moving semi-truck flatbed, I picked up bales and tossed them onto the truck. Someone did the same thing on the other side. It was Phil's job to stack the bales on the truck.

When they were dry, bales weighed around 30 pounds. When they were wet, they seemed to weigh a ton. My legs were in pretty good shape at this time, but this was backbreaking work. By lunchtime, I was limping noticeably. The boss-man informed everyone that in the afternoon I would drive.

I had to remind the morning driver of that when we got back to the truck. He got out from behind the wheel, but he was so mad at me that he threatened to beat me up. He swore at me all afternoon. Phil and the other loader reminded him that we were out there to haul bales, not fight. That's when he announced that he would get me after work, at night.

It wasn't like we could lock him out. The bunkhouse garage had no doors. We'd have to keep watch through the starlit night. Phil had a .22 revolver, something he'd bought a few weeks earlier from another "cowboy." He kept the loaded gun under his pillow that night. We moved our cots close together so that either of us could grab it if it became necessary. The angry driver didn't show, fortunately.

The job had other "Wild West" aspects, too, including riding a horse for the first time. I'd never done more than sit on top of a sturdy plow horse and suddenly I was learning how to throw a saddle on a mustang and cinch it up.

The ranch had 900 head of cattle. As each 3,000-acre section of field was harvested, they had to be herded onto it to graze on the remaining grass and straw. First, though, we had to round them up on the 5,000-acre pasture on which they'd spent part of the summer.

I was assigned a 20-year-old horse named Tex, a cutting horse who was so experienced he almost didn't need me. He could keep a group of skittish cattle in a single file line or separate a cow or calf from the herd if you hinted at which one you wanted. It was a pure delight working with Tex. I came to really respect and trust him. I think he felt the same about me. On one occasion, anyway, I got him to step over a section of downed barbed wire fence rather than go 200 yards around it. The experienced cowhands who saw it said that Tex had never done that before.

By mid-September, the harvest was done and we'd completed all the related chores. A few regulars stayed, but most of us headed home.

Back at the U, I found an apartment with one of my new friends from Montana, a guy who had come to the Twin Cities to study radio announcing. It was on University Avenue, just 10 blocks from campus, but on the opposite side from the hospital. I could have taken the bus to campus, but instead I rode a bicycle. It probably saved a few dollars in bus fare, but it cost a lot more in the long term. It made it too easy to skip class or avoid tests when it was cold or snowy. I missed classes when I was on campus, too: Time would get away from me somehow and I'd simply forget to go. I flunked differential equations, a required class, when I erroneously decided that I didn't have to attend because the course was being replaced with a different one the next quarter. Wrong. I was enrolled in it, and it still counted.

In spring, I moved into a rented house with Jim and Jack, from the Walnut Street rooming house, and four other students. It hadn't occurred to me to look the brothers up when I returned to the university the previous fall. I'd never had long-term friends outside of Gillette and had no idea what you had to do to keep friendships going. I was surprised when, after a chance meeting on campus, they asked me where I'd disappeared to, and I was flattered when they asked me to share the house with them.

It wasn't the smartest choice I could have made. With my academic life going into an all-too-familiar downward spiral, I was becoming desperate for social distractions, for anything except coursework. When any one of the six others in the house didn't study, I decided I didn't need to either. They were my role models, unfortunately, not the ones who were studying, who were invisible to me.

I found a second job to supplement my earnings at the food service. Pillsbury Mills, on Washington Avenue, was looking for a night watchman. After a short conversation, the interviewer asked me if I had ever shot a gun.

"Sure," I responded. "I grew up on a farm with rifles and shotguns."

He hired me and handed me a pistol to carry while on guard duty. The first night someone gave me a clock box and showed me how to insert into it the keys that were hung along the route in order to record my visits to each location. He didn't tell me, though, what I was supposed to be watching for. I didn't have a radio, so if I saw something strange I'd have to run to the phone in the guard shack and try to call the dispatcher.

I had to do rounds every hour. I had intended to study in between the half-hour-long circuits, but my books rarely got opened after I started resting for 10 or 15 minutes after every trip.

Days and nights started getting mixed up. I was always tired, always had an excuse for napping instead of going to class. I missed tests.

My social life also suffered. I couldn't justify going out with a friend when things were going so badly in class. I didn't study instead of socializing, of course. I just worried about studying.

Finally, I got a letter from the U that said I was not making satisfactory progress and should stop in to see a counselor. I went as instructed and he suggested that I take a year or two off. I agreed with him—I could not continue as I had the previous two quarters.

I dropped all my classes, but kept the two jobs in order to support myself. The food service job wouldn't last much longer, I knew; it was only for students.

A few days later, Mother and Dad drove up to the house. I invited them into my room, which was in its usual good order. It was hard to be too messy when you didn't have many belongings.

"Hi, what are you doing here?" I asked.

They had received a letter from the U about my progress, they said, and they were thinking it might be a good idea if I just came home to sort everything out. I agreed, and they drove back to Watkins.

I quit my jobs, packed my stuff into the car, and drove home the next day. This time I did not say good-bye to anyone.

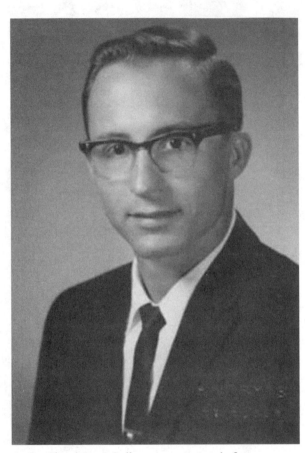

At St. Cloud State College, in 1963, just before
student teaching

*a*fter I'd been at home a month, helping with the chores but otherwise not doing much of anything or going anywhere, Dad decided to speak up.

"What do you plan to do?" he asked. "You can't go on the way you have the last few years."

"Well, at least I'm not in jail," I responded. I don't think he was amused.

Work. Eat. Sleep. Think. Work. Eat. Sleep. Think. Work . . .

I decided that this must be what it was like to be a monk. I also decided that I did not want to spend the rest of my life that way.

I knew where the problem lay, unfortunately. I had nobody to blame but myself.

I was an adult. Most of the members of my high school class who'd gone to college had graduated the year before and were starting careers.

My legs were fixed for all practical purposes: I hadn't had an operation since 1955, and after examinations in the spring of 1957 and 1959, Dr. Babb had concluded that "no further treatment is indicated at the present time . . ."

I didn't owe anyone any money, but I didn't have real prospects for earning any, either.

I had no friends, though I had met some people who might be friends if only I knew how to make and sustain such relationships.

I was an outside observer of the world, not really part of it. I was just going through the motions, just existing.

I continued in that vein for the better part of a year.

Finally, early in 1963, I came up with a plan that I thought was good enough to share with Dad. I would transfer the quarter credits I'd earned at the University of Minnesota and maybe some of the ones from St. John's and enroll spring quarter at St. Cloud State College, only 23 miles away. I would live at home, help with chores, and drive every day to school.

Dad suggested I set up a study area in my large bedroom above the kitchen. If I studied when I was home, he said, I wouldn't have to help him with the regular daily outside chores like the milking, feeding the cows and hogs, and cleaning the barns. Things could continue that way as long as I kept my grades up.

I visited the State Vocational Rehabilitation Office in St. Cloud. As part of a state program to help crippled children become productive citizens, vocational rehab had paid my tuition while I was at St. John's. To my embarrassment, I hadn't even thought to ask for that aid when I went to the U. Was I still eligible? Yes, the staff said. The state would pick up tuition for a total of up to four years.

Mother and Dad were going to cover fees and the cost of books. I wasn't going to be part of the college social scene, I had decided, so I wouldn't need any money for that. I didn't need to party. I needed to get an education and graduate.

I was shocked when I returned to the classroom that spring. As incompetent as I felt sometimes, when I looked around I could see that most of the students around me were even less prepared, less mature. I was 24, but I felt decades older in comparison. I knew what happened if you did not pay attention in class or if you skipped classes and homework. I had learned more than I thought from my experiences. At least I hoped so.

Being at home helped, too. The sounds of the cows, hogs, and roosters outside my window, though familiar and comforting to a degree, provided constant reminders of the unrelenting work that was required to take care of them. Completing my assignments was child's play compared to milking, shoveling out the hog pens, or doing other chores in sub-zero temperatures.

It really was like starting college life all over, but this time with an advantage, instead of a disadvantage. I was relaxed, instead of anxious or intimidated. All the classes seemed interesting, even the required ones. I knew what I needed to do to succeed in each one and how to do it. I was confident.

I began at St. Cloud with the intention of majoring in physics and minoring in mathematics. I quickly noticed that I was taking the same math courses as the math majors were, that all of my physics classes looked like math classes—and that math majors did not have to write lab reports. I switched to a math major and a physics minor.

Dr. Philip Youngner, my advisor, approved the change. The chair of the department, he taught most of the physics courses I took. He was, hands down, the best teacher I ever had. He'd taught elementary classes for a few years before going on to get his Ph.D. in physics, and it showed. He could make anything understandable and interesting.

It was easy to get to know the instructors at St. Cloud. The math and physics classes were much smaller than those at St. John's and the U, with just 15 to 18 students in them. It was easy meeting other math and physics students, too. We saw each other again and again in our classes.

One of the students I ran into frequently was Lyle Jordan. He became a good friend. We often compared math homework notes. We took our first computer classes together. He was a farm boy like me. Like many of our classmates, he was interested in becoming a math teacher.

I was thinking a lot about teaching at this time. We had a bookcase at home full of old books signed by my grandfather, John A. Maus, a retired elementary school teacher. I enjoyed sharing what I knew and was comfortable around youngsters. If I went into teaching, I could continue studying the math and science I enjoyed. My legs shouldn't be a handicap either.

I would be a teacher, I decided. I had been searching long enough.

In the fall of 1963, I had to indicate where I wanted to do my student teaching. I listed Robbinsdale as my first choice. I was familiar with the outside of the high school from my trips to Gillette. The large building on 42nd Avenue North, also known as Highway 55, was one of the landmarks on our trips to and from the hospital.

Distracted that autumn by my preparations for student teaching, I fell back into a bad habit: I tried to "wing" a physics test. I got a D.

Dr. Youngner asked to see me in the hall after class.

"Where do you think you're going with that D?" he demanded.

A relative had died the week before, I explained. That was true, but it hadn't been the cause of my poor performance. I just hadn't studied.

Dr. Youngner said he couldn't approve me for student teaching the next quarter, not with progress like that.

I told him I thought he was being too severe. After all, this was the first time I had slipped up in his class.

Dr. Youngner offered to allow me to take a different version of the same test three days later, on Monday.

I spent the whole weekend studying, anxious to prove to him that I knew the material, anxious to redeem myself. I took the test in his office, under his watchful eye. I did well, and he signed off on my student teaching.

After Dr. Youngner's wake-up call, I never slacked on physics—or any other class, for that matter. Although he was the first teacher I could remember to confront me about declining performance, I wanted him to be the last.

When I was assigned to student teach at Hosterman Junior High, a new school in Robbinsdale, I rented a room on Broadway Avenue near downtown. My time in the rooming house was almost as instructive as my time in the classroom. My landlord had the most amazing, fantastically clean, and well organized machine shop in the basement of the house. In it he made small brass parts for top-secret nuclear submarines. It was fascinating work. I decided to explore becoming a machinist if teaching didn't pan out.

My mentors at Hosterman were experienced math and science teachers. The students were great. I enjoyed the work and I did it well. So well, in fact, that the principal, Jim Andress, asked me on three different occasions if I wanted to teach at the school in the fall of the following year. I had to explain each time that I was very interested, but I would not be graduating until the first part of 1965.

I returned to St. Cloud for spring quarter in great spirits. My days were spent looking forward in anticipation now, instead of backward in regret. Things were beginning to come together.

What was an airplane doing on the lawn in front of the administration building? Other students were streaming past it, seemingly oblivious to its presence, but the sight stopped me in my tracks.

"How did this get here?" I asked the student sitting at a nearby table.

He was a member of the college's Flying Saints Aero Club, he explained. They'd hauled it in on a trailer after taking out a few bolts and removing the wing. By the next day, it would be back at the St. Cloud Airport and flying again.

Handing me a brochure that promoted the flying club, he mentioned that the faculty advisor to the club was the chair of the math department. Dr. Anderson was also my academic advisor now that I was a math major. I met with him every quarter to talk about course registration and how things were going. I went in and asked him for more information about the club.

The group was always looking for members, I learned. Their three planes flew nearly all day, every day. Members could rent a plane for $3 an hour "wet" (including gas and oil). Hiring an instructor cost another $3 per hour. That was a fraction of the cost anywhere else.

In my hospital bed years earlier, books on flying had introduced me to the joys of reading and libraries. Pictures of planes and the history of aviation had entertained me for hours. I had spent weeks building model airplanes like the B-24 Liberator and the P-51 Mustang. I had flown them in my imagination even longer than that.

I had to do this. The plane on the lawn at the college was the first one I'd ever seen up close. I'd never been inside one, never flown anywhere. I just knew I had to fly or die trying.

I could tell anyone who pressed me that learning to fly was a very practical thing. It tied in with teaching about the physics of flight. It would give me a special skill. It would continue to build my confidence.

On the other hand, it would also cost money. Money that I didn't have.

On the way home I stopped in to see the local banker in Watkins. I was going to need about $300 for flying lessons. Unfortunately, I already had a $400 loan on the car that I had bought to get around when I was student teaching.

"No problem," he said. "We'll just add it to your car loan. You can start payments when you get your first job after you graduate."

His quick response was gratifying. It was nice to know that I wasn't the only one anticipating my graduation. The circle of people who were confident that I was going to finish college, that I was going to get a job, was growing slowly but steadily.

I told Dad when I got home that afternoon that I wanted to take flying lessons over the summer.

"You'll need money," he replied.

"Banks loan money for things like that," I answered. I waited to hear how he felt about me incurring more debt.

"What bank would loan you money for flying," he responded, "especially when you don't have a job?"

I had to explain, then, that I had checked at the bank in town and that everything was set. Dad was surprised, I think. He had never borrowed money for anything that wasn't essential. He gave me the go-ahead, though. Flying wasn't important to him, but he could see that learning to fly was something that I really wanted and needed.

I was looking forward to graduating. It would mark the beginning of a new life, a normal life. Graduating meant I had to make some big decisions, too. I could go to a school somewhere that needed someone to teach the balance of the year, or I could stay and begin graduate courses.

I wanted to finish a second major in physics, and I intended eventually to get a master's degree in mathematics education. I decided to stay in school and start my graduate studies.

Staying on campus would also enable me to stay in touch with the college placement office and watch for fall teaching positions.

I had learned while I was student teaching that in the large suburban schools new teachers usually started in the junior highs, where they taught five classes of the same subject, and then worked their way to the senior highs. Smaller, out-state schools had openings at the high school level; teachers moved up by relocating to large metropolitan schools.

I had a bachelor's degree and was working on a master's. I was 26. I was ready for a real job. After interviewing for schools in Nevada and Illinois, mainly for practice, I spotted an ad from Pine Island, Minnesota.

Where was Pine Island? How far away was it? I did a little research.

Pine Island was a small farming community like Watkins, but located near the cosmopolitan city of Rochester, home to the Mayo Clinic and a division of IBM. In fact, it was becoming a bedroom community for Rochester. The senior high school was looking for someone to teach elective classes in math and physics. The situation looked promising, almost perfect, in fact.

The superintendent gave me a tour of the school and explained which classes they wanted me to teach. They wanted me to be the audiovisual director, too. I said I was interested—and he offered me the job on the spot, at the annual salary paid to all beginning teachers, $4,900. I accepted.

I began my aviation education by enrolling in a summer session class that Dr. Anderson, the flying club advisor, was teaching. Some of the students were elementary classroom teachers working on future lesson plans that revolved around aviation. Five of us, though, were preparing for the written FAA test for the private pilot's license.

In the course of the class, we flew to Memphis in an Air National Guard C-119 cargo plane. The trip in the lumbering boxcar of a plane was interesting, but nothing like the very first time I flew—on July 16, 1965, during my first flying lesson.

That flight, in an agile Aeronca 7EC Champ, was simply the single most exciting thing I'd done in my entire life, easily topping the exhilaration I felt when I helped pull down the old silo or climbed the rope to the top of the barn. I was hooked, especially when I discovered that my legs were more than up to the task of operating the pedals that moved the rudder side to side. It took only a nudge now and then to keep the ball centered in the Turn and Bank Indicator and the plane on a steady, even course.

A few weeks before I was due in Pine Island, I passed the FAA's written pilot's license test. On August 26, after telling me to stop at the end of the runway, my instructor, Richard Latterell, got out of the yellow Champ we'd been practicing in and told me he thought I was ready to solo. I was a bit shocked—I'd completed just a little bit more than the minimum hours of instruction (eight) that were required—but I agreed.

I guided the plane through the mandatory three takeoffs and land-ings, stopping between each for a briefing from my instructor. The first trip was fairly proficient. During the second, I forgot to hold the tail down and the plane bounced a few times. The third time, though, was close to perfect.

I was flying—minus an aircraft—for days afterwards. I had achieved one of my childhood dreams. I was ready for Pine Island, ready to take the next step in my journey.

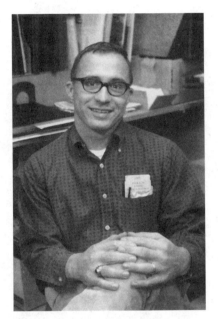

During my second year teaching
math and physics in Pine Island,
Minnesota

*M*y first class of the day in Pine Island had just three students in it. They were taking advanced math in preparation for attending college the following year. It was followed by two sections of trigonometry and a physics class. The day ended with a course on plane geometry. In addition, I oversaw the audiovisual department, making sure the filmstrip projectors, overhead projectors, and tape recorders were in working order and where they needed to be at any given time.

Five elective classes with a total of 68 students, or fewer than 14 students per class on average: It was a dream schedule.

Pine Island High School served students in grades 7 through 12. The staff was small and relatively young. There were a few old-timers around who could tell stories of the early days, but three-fourths of the faculty had been teaching no more than five years. In the fall of 1965 nine of us were new to the school.

I hadn't asked much about the social aspects of the job when I'd accepted it, but I should have. After all, life in Pine Island could have been very dull or horribly lonesome.

As it turned out, it was neither. It was easy to get involved in the life of the school. In fact, it was almost inescapable. Teachers sold tickets at afternoon and evening athletic events and supervised dances, meetings of student clubs, and anything else that happened after school.

Socializing with other teachers was also nearly mandatory. By the end of the last period of the school day, everyone had an invitation to get together and knew when and where they were to meet. By the end of the football game, you even knew who would be riding with whom.

Even if I'd wanted to, and I definitely didn't, it would have been almost impossible to get out of participating without seeming anti-social. Forsaking my loner ways, I joined the young, single faculty when they gathered at a bar in a neighboring town or at the apartment of two gregarious young women, Dorothy Jacoby, a music teacher, and Donna Hobson, who taught science, health, and physical education. Their place was the *de facto* after-school teachers' lounge. Sometimes there were five of us there, other times 15.

I was too busy to dwell on the problems of my past. When students and staff inquired about my slight limp, I told them I'd had polio, but little more. It was like being able to hit the RESET button at the bowling alley or on a pinball machine. Pine Island was a whole new game for me.

I had the best teaching job I could imagine and a social life to match it. Could life get any better?, I wondered.

One day in early fall the principal came to my room during class. Pulling me aside, he asked if I could come down to the office to take a call from my dad. I was alarmed. Something horrible must have happened to cause Dad to phone me, especially while I was at work.

I needn't have worried, as it turned out. Dad was calling because his brother Johnny was not going to be able to drive because of declining health and he was giving me the first chance to buy his '63 Plymouth. It was just two years old and had only about 12,000 miles on it.

"I'd love to," I told Dad, "but how am I going to pay for it? I have two loans on the car I'm driving and still haven't made a payment."

"I already talked to the bank," Dad said, "and they can combine all three loans on this car."

I told him to set things up. The car, my fourth, was the first one to have less than a hundred thousand miles on it when I purchased it. My universe was starting to get into balance.

I couldn't say the same thing about my bank balance. I was barely making ends meet.

Knowing that new teachers always arrived poor, the school district paid them half of their September check on the 15th. I'd get the second half on September 30—but it would have to last until the end of October.

When I looked at the check at the end of the month, I was shocked.

"Why is this so small?" I asked the bookkeeper behind the front office counter.

"The deductions for the month are all taken out at the end of the month," she explained. "For everybody."

I managed to borrow a few hundred at the local bank. It would get me through October, but having to take out a loan gave me pause. I wasn't a big spender. I was renting an inexpensive room at Mrs. Hart's house. I rarely had breakfast and I ate lunch in the school cafeteria and dinner at the Rainbow Café, an inexpensive diner. Something was off, I decided, if I had to go into hock to get through the second month on the job.

I had hoped never again to wear a cast or use crutches, but fate gave me another chance in October when I went horseback riding with a student.

His mother warned me that my horse was a jumper and that I needed to be careful. I didn't pay much attention. I didn't expect to be jumping anything, and besides, I had ridden horses in Montana, herding cattle.

We were galloping through a pair of gates in the fence surrounding an open pasture. The horse and I simultaneously noticed that the third fence-gate, made of barbed wire, was closed. He slid on all four legs; I thought for sure that we were going to roll and crash through the gate. I slipped to one side, preparing to jump off if the horse hit the fence.

It was just about then that he made a big graceful leap up and over the fence. I was riding an air-saddle. I landed on the ground, scattered rocks all around me. The horse stood there, looking down at me and wondering, probably, why I had abandoned ship.

My ankle hurt a little, but the pain was manageable. I got back on the horse, and we returned to the barn.

By Sunday, the ankle hurt so much that I couldn't walk on it. I'd been invited to dinner at Donna and Dorothy's. After I called to say I wasn't going to be able to make it, Donna brought dinner to my room at the boardinghouse. The meals on wheels-type offering included rolls burned to a charcoal-like consistency. I was grateful for the food—and a bit astonished that anyone would go to that kind of trouble for me.

On Monday the pain was so bad that instead of going to school, I went to Saint Marys Hospital in Rochester. An x-ray showed a crack in an anklebone of the right foot. The doctor wrapped my leg in a cast and sent me home.

By Wednesday, I was once again in a high school classroom encased in plaster and encumbered by crutches. I was a little unsettled by how much at home I felt in the situation. I used to hate being different, being disabled. This time, though, it was fun, not frustrating.

For one thing, I knew my condition was a temporary one.

For another thing, I was enjoying showing off my skills. The students and staff could see that I was very proficient with the crutches. They were impressed by the crossover; they'd never seen it before. They talked easily about my polio and without looking at me like I was some kind of victim.

Another of my childhood wishes had been granted, I realized. I finally had a glamorous reason to have a cast on my leg. Until it came off in six weeks, I could regale people with the tale of the colorful way that I had acquired it.

The school had a Van de Graf generator, but it was a mess. One early winter evening I went in to repair it. It took some work, but eventually the apparatus was once again producing static lightning-bolt electrical sparks nearly a foot long between its two large aluminum spheres.

I was about to shut it down and go home when I heard a noise. To my surprise, in walked Donna Hobson. She'd come to the school to get something, she said. When she saw my car out front, she'd decided to come to the science lab to see what I was up to.

I showed her what I was going to do with the students in physics the next day. I connected her to the sparking globes. She became a million-volt conductor. Her electrically charged hair radiated straight out from her head. She might have been scared, but she didn't show it.

She had a great sense of adventure, I thought, as well as a wonderful way of making people feel so at home that they felt comfortable falling asleep on her couch. I wondered if that was because of her upbringing. Her parents, Dolford and Alice Hobson, ran a restaurant in Cleveland, Minnesota, she'd told me, and they lived in back of it until she was 11. She literally grew up in public. It was hard to picture what that must have been like. It was so different from the solitary existence of my child-hood, spent roaming the farm with my dog or in a hospital bed with a book or an airplane model.

I went home for the holidays. On New Year's Day, I helped Dad slaughter and quarter a steer that had broken its hip on the ice the night before. We talked a little as we worked.

It looked to him like I liked my job in Pine Island, he said.

Yes, I replied. It felt like things were finally going well in my life, I told him.

They *were* going well. I was enjoying life as a first-year teacher and enjoying getting to know Donna better. The group continued to go to Rochester for concerts and dining out. Once or twice she and I ended up doing something together, like listening to her Jim Reeves' LPs. She just might be right for me, I thought, if she liked music like that.

On March 17, a major snowstorm hit southern Minnesota, and school was canceled for three days. We had one long party. Donna and I decided during the break that we wanted to get married. We announced our engagement to the staff when school resumed. Everyone was sur-prised. In fact, when Donna told one friend, "I'm going to marry Richard," she replied, "Richard who?"

Next we told our parents.

I told Mother and Dad over Sunday dinner. They were a little sur-prised, too, but accepting. They'd also gotten to know each other prima-rily through group social activities and when they decided to get married did so fairly quickly, less than a month after the banns were first read in church. They looked forward to meeting Donna, they said.

Donna had a slightly tougher time with her parents. She was just two years out of college, and they thought she should wait a while before making this kind of commitment. Her father's resistance crumbled, though, when he heard I was working on my private pilot's license. In his younger days, he and his pals had often hunted foxes from a low-flying plane. He decided that if I could also fly a plane, I was okay. I had yet another reason to be grateful that I'd noticed that airplane on campus that day and joined the flying club.

We set a date for the wedding: August 27, 1966.

In the spring, I was recruited to play baseball.

As I noted earlier, in a school the size of the one in Pine Island everyone—students and staff alike—gets recruited for everything. Every activity needs more participants.

Coaches get particularly adept at finding the bodies they need. A wrestling coach, for instance, might tell a student that basketball was bad for him so he'd go out for wrestling instead. Or a baseball coach might fill out the faculty squad by twisting the arm of a science teacher who'd had polio.

That's what happened to me. Between classes, Coach Gannon stuck his head into my room. "Hey, Maus. We need you. The student-faculty game is next Tuesday. You can make it, can't you?"

"I haven't actually played much baseball," I replied. "I don't even watch it very often."

"No problem," he said. "We've got some power players; half the team is coaches. If we can't field nine players, though, we're dead in the water. We'll have to forfeit. We can't make it without you."

Before he dashed off, he said, "Don't worry. You'll do fine."

What, me worry? Just because I hadn't played the game since grade school and most of my teammates were going to be lifelong athletes? Of course I wasn't worried. I was petrified.

The day after the game, the students came into my classroom, stared at me, and shook their heads. They asked if I had played baseball before I got polio. I told them I contracted polio when I was a baby.

They could not believe what I'd done—and neither could I: In the big game the afternoon before, facing the varsity team's star pitcher, I'd gotten three hits in three at bats. Each time, I drove the ball into the out-field, right over the first baseman's head, and easily reached base. Nobody, student or faculty, did better.

In the teachers' lounge, the coaches gave me a good ribbing: "Hey, Maus, I thought you couldn't run."

"I usually can't," I replied, "but it was easy on that thin layer of sand between home and first."

The base path had felt just like the tobacco-shed road, as a matter of fact. I felt like I had wings as I raced down it.

I did the math. Counting only games with umpires, where at least one team wore uniforms, I had a lifetime batting average of one thousand.

Trips to Rochester, Watkins, and Donna's hometown, Cleveland, made the rest of the spring pass quickly. I attended summer school at St. Cloud State College, where I worked on my master's degree and resumed my flying lessons. Most weekends I drove from Watkins to Cleveland to be with Donna. We spent many sunny afternoons on the shores of Lake Jefferson.

In August, Donna and I were married and I moved into her apartment, replacing Dorothy, who got married shortly thereafter herself.

During my second year in Pine Island, I was elected president of the Pine Island Education Association. I'd been fairly vocal as a first-year

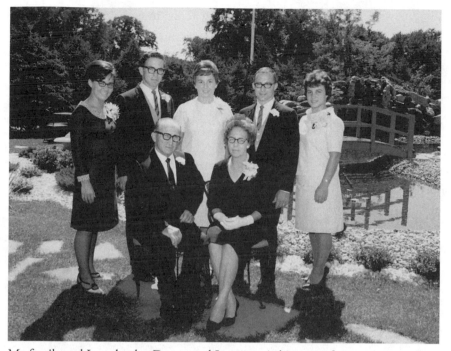

My family and I on the day Donna and I got married in 1966: front row, my parents, Benno and Lorrayne Maus; back row, Louise, Phil, Ruth, me, and Helen

teacher, and the faculty knew that I wasn't afraid to speak up. I also volunteered, with the group's support, to serve as the salary negotiator.

It was an interesting, fast-moving year. Now that I wasn't scrambling to figure out what to do in class every day, I began to hone my teaching skills, began to reflect on what helped people succeed, in the classroom and outside of it.

Living and working in Pine Island had transformed my life. I'd found it easy here to join in activities, to meet and make friends. Part of that, I knew, could be attributed to the fact that it is almost impossible not to participate in things in a small town or a small school.

So why had it been so difficult for me in Watkins? I hadn't been ready, I think, and there was no one to help me get ready. In the 1940s, 50s, and 60s, people were just beginning to realize how intertwined our physical and psychological states are. My parents, teachers, and doctors never understood, I think, how difficult it was for me to have two almost entirely separate existences, a Watkins one and a hospital one. And I never understood that I didn't have to make it entirely on my own, that additional academic and emotional help might be available if I could find a way to ask for it.

What I was coming to understand about my own childhood and adolescence had a big influence on my teaching. For one thing, I found myself keeping an eye out for the quiet kids on the fringes. For another, I assigned homework and expected that students do it, but homework was much less important to me than it had been to my high school teachers.

I also became an advocate for extracurricular activities, especially non-athletic ones, that were effective in drawing in students and providing them with rewarding skills and social contact. I re-activated the school's camera club. The students took yearbook pictures, developed the films, and printed the pictures in the school darkroom.

I continued developing my own skills as well. During one incredible week in the summer of 1967, I took the written test for my master's degree and the FAA flight test for my private license. I passed both. In my "spare time" that week, I also did all the course work for a two-credit, special arrangement physics course and completed my major in physics.

In the spring of 1968, the end of my third year at Pine Island, I applied for a job in Robbinsdale, where I had done my student teaching. When I didn't receive a reply, Robbinsdale teacher Lee Jordan, wife of my friend Lyle Jordan, suggested that I call the personnel director. There was a general impression that he gave priority to applicants who took that kind of initiative. It turned out that the personnel director was Jim Andress, the former principal at Hosterman Junior High and the man who had offered me a job three times when I was student teaching there.

Before I could call for an interview, though, it was April 15. The school superintendent in Pine Island had given us the impression that teachers who intended to leave had to give notice by that date. Donna and I were expecting our first child and I didn't have another job lined up—but we submitted our resignations anyway. It seemed likely that I would be able to get something in the Robbinsdale area. If not—well, I was optimistic that I'd find something else.

Happily, I didn't have to find an alternative. I interviewed in Robbinsdale and got the job. Beginning in the fall of 1968, I would teach seventh and eighth grade math at Plymouth Junior High School.

As Donna and I left Pine Island at the end of the 1967-68 school year, I couldn't help but think back to the awkward departure from St. John's and to leaving the U without a single good-bye or backward glance. This leave-taking was such a far cry from the dark days when I thought I'd never have a life worth living. I didn't doubt that there would be plenty of challenges ahead of me in the years to come—but I knew there'd be plenty of rewards, too. I'd made it past the biggest hurdles, past the polio and the despair. The path ahead was bright and full of promise.

Epilogue

I truly feel I was lucky as a child.

I was lucky to have a supportive family. I was lucky that I wasn't more severely affected when I contracted polio. I was lucky to receive care in a hospital designed for children just like me.

I was lucky to go to a small school with extracurricular opportunities like band and camera club. Lucky to have the unconditional love of a dog like Rex and a farm to explore with him. Lucky to discover books and, through them, ways to explore the world and the universe.

When undiagnosed and untreated clinical childhood depression led to thoughts of suicide, I was lucky to be able to find reasons to go on living.

When rage led me to contemplate ways to put a stop to wrongs that I felt had been done to me, I was lucky to find a way to avoid a tragedy like the shootings that occurred at Red Lake High School and Rocori High School in Minnesota and Columbine in Colorado.

I am also lucky because, after retirement, I found a therapist familiar with Post-Traumatic Stress Disorder who helped me begin to come to terms with some of the most difficult aspects of my childhood. I am lucky to have been able to continue the healing process by writing this memoir.

I am sure that in reading my story there were times when you, like I, scratched your head and wondered, "What *were* they thinking?" Or "How could anyone have *ever* thought that was the right thing to do?" Or "Why didn't anybody see how crucial it was to do something about that situation right then and there?"

All of which prompts me to ask, "What are we doing—or not doing—today that will cause people in 50 years to say the same things about us?"

FACT: Polio has yet to be eliminated, despite the availability of an effective vaccine.

The number of polio cases has been reduced from 350,000 in 1988 to around 1,350 in 2005, according to the Global Polio Eradication Initiative. This is a coalition of the World Health Organization, the U.S. Centers for Disease Control and Prevention, UNICEF, and Rotary International, the service organization committed to the noble goal of achieving a polio-free world.

The progress that has been made to date is impressive, but we need to do even more. Six countries remain polio endemic (Nigeria, India, Pakistan, Afghanistan, Niger, and Egypt). Ten previously polio-free countries have been re-infected (Somalia, Indonesia, Yemen, Angola, Ethiopia, Chad, Sudan, Mali, Eritrea, and Cameroon).

We in the United States can't be complacent, either. In the fall of 2005, five cases of polio were reported—among un-inoculated children in southern Minnesota. We need to make sure that never happens again anywhere in this country.

FACT: The third leading cause of death among teens and young adults is suicide, according to the National Mental Health Association. Nearly 80 percent of children and teens who need mental health services don't receive them, the NMHA says. Each year almost 5,000 people ages 15 to 24 kill themselves.

Young people in the U.S. are being crippled today by things that are every bit as severe as polio was in my youth. They are being cut off from full participation in life by depression and other mental illness. By addictions. By bullying and harassment. By disabilities. By language and cultural difference. By poverty and homelessness. By physical, sexual, and psychological abuse. By families that are dysfunctional—and by a foster care system that sometimes can be equally disruptive to their lives and well being.

We can't fix everything. Progress won't happen overnight. The good news is that these conditions are as capable of being redressed as polio is.

Every child deserves someone who cares. Consider being that person. Having a healthy, happy childhood and life shouldn't be a matter of getting lucky.

For more information on polio, teen mental health, and other issues and ways you can be involved in addressing them, see the Internet links at www.luckyonebook.com.

Apple Crunch Recipe

I copied this recipe down by hand a half century ago and have it still. I fondly remember the first time I made the dish—because I made it all by myself. The teacher in the Gillette classroom/kitchen answered a few questions for me, but nobody helped me peel, cut, measure, or stir. I put the apple crunch in the oven on my own, watched the time, and took it out. It smelled so good. We ate the treat with a little cream on it while it was still warm. (Today I would recommend ice cream.) I invite you to help a youngster have this same wonderful experience.

4 c	tart apples	1 c	brown sugar—divided
½ c	water	1 c	cornflakes crunched
1 tsp	cinnamon	½ c	butter

Peal and slice the apples. Arrange them in a greased casserole. Pour the water over them. Sprinkle the cinnamon and ½ c brown sugar over the apples.

Place the crushed cornflakes in a bowl and add ½ c brown sugar and the melted butter. Stir, and then spread the mixture over the apples. Pack it firmly with a spoon.

Bake at 350° until the apples are tender and the crust is brown. This will take about 30 minutes.

Serve with cream or lemon sauce.

Glossary

ANTERIOR: Located on or near the front of the body

ATROPINE SULPHATE: Medication for drying of secretions

ATROPHY: Decrease in size of body tissue, or part

CODEINE SULPHATE: Painkiller, derived from morphine

DISTAL: Situated away from point of attachment

EPIPHYSEAL ARREST: Staples across epiphyseal to halt expansion

EPIPHYSEAL PLATE: Disk of cartilage where bone growth occurs

GENU VALGUS: Knock-knee condition

IATROGENIC: Physician-induced harm

LAMBRINUDI: Operation using staples to prevent foot drop

LATERAL: On the side, away from the middle

MEDIAL: On the side, toward the middle

MORPHINE: Most effective painkiller

OPERATION: Synonym for surgery

ORTHOPEDIC: Relating to skeleton, joints, and ligaments

OSTEOTOMY: Surgical division or sectioning of bone

POLIOMYELITIS: Infectious disease caused by the poliovirus

POSTERIOR: Toward the hind part of the body

Chronology of Hospitalizations and Treatments

Admit	Days	Operation	Date	Procedure
1	314		1939–1940	Posterior splint, right foot
2	85	1	4-24-1944	Open lengthening of tendo Achiles, right
3	164	2	1-16-1950	Lambrinudi, right foot; staple epiphyseal plates left knee
3		3	3-20-1950	Flexion contracture of left knee
3		4	5-09-1950	Extend left knee, apply stovepipe cast
4	38	5	7-17-1951	Posterior bone block, right astragalus
5	89	6	4-01-1952	Posterior bone block, right astragalus, bone from left anterior tibia
6	86	7	7-08-1952	Explore draining sinus, right heel
6		8	7-14-1952	Delayed primary closure of wound, right heel
6		9	9-02-1952	Excision of scar over Achilles tendon, right
7	44	10	1-13-1953	Remove staples, lateral femoralepiphysis; remove and replace medial

Admit	Days	Operation	Date	Procedure
8	39	11	10-13-1953	Remove staples, medial epicondyle; Phemister operation
9	66	12	7-19-1955	Supracondylar osteotomy, left femur
9		13	7-28-1955	Insertion of Steinman pin, proximal end of left tibia
9		14	8-04-1955	Insertion of Kirchner wire, distal end of left femur
9		15	8-05-1955	Manipulation of left knee under anesthetic
9		16	8-16-1955	Open reduction and internal fixation, left femur—attach plate and 4 screws
10	13		9-19-1955	Replace broken cast

938   Total
93.8   Average

(A full-time nurse would work about 11 years to accumulate 938 days in the hospital.)

The Medical Records

Verbatim excerpts from the files of Gillette State Hospital for Crippled Children for patient Richard A. Maus, 1939-1959.

Chapter 1

ADMISSION #1

11-2-1939 (HISTORY)
About August 20, 1939, the patient became rather acutely ill, and for three days he was very irritable. During this time he had a severe upper respiratory infection, and cried when he was touched. After a few days the acute illness subsided.
Referred by: Dr. A. Mahowald, Albany, Minnesota

11-2-1939
Family history negative for orthopedic abnormalities, tuberculosis, cancer, and diabetes. No operations and no injuries.
Diagnosis on admission – Residual Poliomyelitis, right foot
(Onset August 20, 1939)

11-2-1939
The patient is a well developed, well nourished child, six months of age. At present in no acute distress.

11-2-1939
In the right leg there is some muscular atrophy due to Poliomyelitis. Patient has, however, still a little motion in the leg.

11-2-1939
Admitted to Ward 2 at 1:30 P.M. Isolated in cubicle. Given routine admission care. Splint applied to right foot as ordered. ...
No teeth.

11-6-1939
Approved for dental work on Tuesday, November 7.

11-9-1939
Smooth splint on the inside. The right foot feels tight. Leave the splint off until his heel is healed.

11-9-1939
Given Pertussis vaccine ... 1 c.c. into each arm, first dose.

11-16-1939
Given Pertussis vaccine ... 1-1/2 c.c. into left arm and thigh.

11-16-1939
Temperature 101.2° at 6:30 P.M. Large discolored area on the left thigh from Pertussis vaccine.

11-17-1939
Temperature 101.6° at 8 A.M. Right heel very red. Splint left off.
Area on left thigh appears better.

11-23-1939
Given Pertussis vaccine 1-1/2 c.c. into left thigh and right arm, third and last dose.

11-28-1939
New long leg plaster applied to right leg as directed.

Neurological examination:As far as can be seen, the fundi are normal. The pupils are equal and regular, and respond promptly to light. Convergence is normal and pupils contract. Facial movements are normal. The patient moves both upper extremities with equal facility. There is no hypertonus on either side. The lower extremities show normal muscle tone. The distal third of the right calf is somewhat smaller than the left. Knee jerks are present, but the left seems somewhat more

active than the right. Ankle jerks are equal. Plantar responses are normal. The right foot is slightly inverted, and there is a shortening of the right tendo Achilles.
DIAGNOSIS: Residual Poliomyelitis, right foot.
Treatment: Orthopedic.

12-5-1939
Cast on right foot has slipped. Plaster bivalved; reddened area over heel. Bivalved plaster reapplied.

12-6-1939
Metal night splint applied to right foot as ordered by Dr. ...

12-21-1939
Do not think that present splint will hold foot.

12-22-1939
Posterior plaster splint made for the right foot.

1-14-1940
Weight 18 pounds. Gained 1 ounce in the past week. Appetite is very good. Is active and happy.

1-18-1940
To have physiotherapy and message to right leg.

4-9-1940
Re-cast model for castex splint is not satisfactory. Another will be made.

4-26-1940
Patient may be transferred to Ward 3. Transferred to Ward III from Ward II. Put on 3 meals a day.

5-5-1940
Weight 19 pounds, 11 ounces. Gaining weight. Eats well. Happy. Plays by himself.

6-16-1940
Appetite is very good. Tries to stand up in bed.

7-7-1940
Is very active. Stands up in his crib. Has two teeth.

7-18-1940
Make plaster model for long leg brace, right. Make splint for the right foot to use at night.

7-25-1940
Long leg brace to be attached to the shoe. Brace to have no joints; use light weight steel.

8-29-1940
Seen walking. Is walking fairly well.

9-5-1940
Discharged improved. ... To wear his short right leg brace during the day; to have a new Castex night splint made, sufficiently long to hold his toes.

9-10-1940
Discharged to mother, Mrs. Benno Maus, at 4:35 P.M. ... Mother instructed regarding exercises, application of brace and splint. Skin in good condition.

DISCHARGE #1

12-16-40
Castex splint made for the right foot over the recast model.

12-19-40
Splint mailed to patient.

3-15-1941
Leg brace mailed to patient.

4-17-1941

The foot is in good position. There is practically no anterior tibial function. To have plaster model made for new castex night splint, right foot. To have new shoes. ... To report in 6 months.

8-28-1941

The right heel is being drawn up by a short heel cord and he has a semi-rocker type of foot. Mother is to apply hot packs to right lower leg. Discontinue the brace, but get him a new metal night splint. To report in three months.

9-23-1941

Shoes built up and mailed.

1-5-1942

In reply to letter from patient's mother stating that his splint did not fit, she was advised to bring him down on a Thursday morning in the near future.

1-6-1942

Shoes built up and mailed.

7-16-1942

The patient walks quite well, but has a foot drop on the right. New shoes are to be built up as follows: Check strap on the right shoe; 1/8-inch lift on the inner aspect of each heel. Shoes to be mailed when completed. To report in six months.

11-19-1942

The right foot cannot be brought up to within 10° or 15° of the right angle, and the foot is pronated. Put in a light spring steel in the sole of the right shoe and build up the inner edge of the heel and sole 1/8 inch, light leather arch in shoe. Continue with the check strap on the right shoe. To report in February or March 1943.

3-1-1943

In reply to letter received from the patients father, letter was dictated advising that it would be all right for patient to report to the St. Cloud clinic.

1943

SEEN AT ST. CLOUD CLINIC:

DIAGNOSIS: Residual Poliomyelitis, right foot.

Apparently, the steel in the right shoe is broken. The shoe should be sent to Gillette to have a new one put in. Continue with the check strap.

7-20-1943

Tonsillectomy and adenoidectomy performed by Dr. Mahowald.

3-25-1944

SEEN AT ST. CLOUD CLINIC:

Diagnosis: Residual Poliomyelitis, right foot.

Mother says patient is walking more on the toes of the right foot, although patient is having no subjective complaints. Examination shows a rather marked contracture of the right calf muscle. The treatment here is very definitely hospitalization with attempts to lengthen posterior structures either by hot packs and physiotherapy, or operation. Should be admitted to the hospital as soon as possible.

ADMISSION #2

4-20-1944

Diagnosis on admission – Contracted tendo Achilles, right side, due to Anterior Poliomyelitis (Onset August 20, 1939)

Length of right leg 48 centimeters; left 52 centimeters. Circumference of right thigh 22 centimeters; left 24-1/2 centimeters. Circumference of right leg 16 centimeters; left 20 centimeters. There is weakness, Grade 1, of the right quadriceps, but useful. Right foot drop with tight shortened tendo Achilles, active posterior tibial, absent anterior tibial and peroneal.

4-23-1944
Approved for surgery; orders written.

4-23-1944
Given Nembutal grains 1/2 at 8 P.M.

4-24-1944 (Author's Note - Fifth Birthday)
Given Nembutal grains 1/2 at 8 A.M.
Atropine grains 1/300, codeine grains 1/2 given 9:10 A.M.
Taken to surgery at 9:40 A.M.

4-24-1944
OPERATION: 4-24-44: Open lengthening of tendo Achilles, right.
Under general anesthesia, an incision approximately 2-inch long was made along the medial side of the right tendo Achilles, and, by dull dissection, the tendon was dissected out of the subcutaneous fat. Anterior-posterior Z plasty was done. The tendon was lengthened enough to bring the foot to just beyond a right angle, and re-sutured with interrupted sutures of chromic catgut. The fascia was closed with plain catgut, and the skin with black silk interrupted sutures. Sterile dressings were applied, followed by plaster of Paris cast extending from the mid thigh to include the toes.

4-24-1944
May have codeine grains 1/2 by hypo. Every 4 hours p.r.n. for pain during the next 48 hours. Elevate the right foot and watch circulation.

4-24-1944
Returned to Ward at 10:50 A.M. in good condition. Right leg elevated. Circulation, sensation, and motion in toes good. Given Codeine grains 1/2 at 2:30 P.M. Slept well during the night. No complaints.

5-6-1944
Remove the cast, right leg, and to have a bandage applied.

5-25-1944
Ace bandage removed. Patient wearing shoes and practicing walking.

7-13-1944
Discharged, improved; to report in October.
Discharged to his aunt at 2 P.M. ... Wearing shoes with check strap on (right) shoe.

DISCHARGE #2

8-30-44
Right shoe built up and Mailed.

10-26-44
The patient still has slight equinus of the right foot, pes planus, and the arch of the shoe should be reinforced with a short steel, and he should have a light leather arch in the shoe. Mother was instructed to continue manipulating the foot every day, and when he gets new shoes to send in the right one to be altered. Patient to report in the spring.

11-8-44
Shoe built up and mailed.

6-7-45
Shoe built up and mailed to patient.

7-11-45
Shoe built up and mailed.

9-13-45
The patient has a new brace on the right leg today, which fits very nicely. Mr. Palm to try to combine the strap of the inside T strap with that of the toe check strap. Also, to have a felt metatarsal pad on the left shoe. To report to the clinic in the spring.

Chapter 2

4-6-46

His general condition is good. No complaints to make except that it is difficult for him to walk in mud or snow. Mother states that in the past there has been a full length steel and the last pair did not have this. She would like to have the new shoes fixed up so there is a full length steel. ... To report in six months.

4-16-46

Shoes built up and mailed to patient--Full length steel in right shoe. Wears an outside iron, inside T. strap. Combine the T with that of the toe check strap; also felt metatarsal pad on the left shoe.

8-22-46

Patient's check strap, outside iron, and inside T strap on the right leg seem to be working satisfactorily. No further recommendations, except to keep this in good repair. This boy will eventually probably have to have a triple arthrodesis. To be seen in about 4 months.

12-12-46

New shoes approved but need the following built up: Full length steel on sole of right shoe, and outside iron and inside T strap with toe-drop check. To have longitudinal arch supports in both shoes. Report to St. Cloud clinic in spring.

12-20-46

Shoes built up and mailed.

1-25-47

Shoes repaired and mailed to patient.

4-2-47

Shoes repaired and mailed to patient.

6-3-47
Shoes repaired and mailed to patient.

9-12-47
Right shoe built up and mailed to patient.

10-13-47
Right shoe built up and mailed to patient.

4-8-48
Shoe built up and mailed to patient.

8-21-48
Brace repaired, shoe built up and mailed to patient.

10-28-48
Right shoe built up and mailed to patient.

11-23-48
Right shoe built up and mailed to patient.

3-19-49
There is about 3/4 of an inch discrepancy leg length and after foot stabilization is done, this will probably be about 1 inch or more. The boy is now 10 years old. Certainly when he is no more than 12 years old consideration should be given for foot stabilization procedure probably of the Lambrinudi type. An epiphyseal arrest the distal end of the left femur can be done at that time.

3-31-49
Shoe built up and mailed to patient.

4-7-49
Right shoe built up and mailed to patient.

9-16-49

Right shoe built up and mailed to patient. Elizabeth McGregor,
Supt.

11-4-49

Right shoe built up and mailed to patient. Jean D. Conklin,
Supt.

Chapter 3

ADMISSION #3

1-5-50
READMITTED.
Patient is a 10-1/2 year old boy not acutely ill.
DIAGNOSIS: Residual poliomyelitis of the right lower extremity.
Upper extremities: No residuals of polio noted.
Lower extremities: The right leg is 1-1/2 inches shorter than
the left. There is involvement of the entire limb, but he has
good quadriceps, good hamstrings and fair triceps surae. There
is some tightness of the iliotibial band. The gluteus medius is
weak.

1-5-50
To be re-admitted. The patient has residual poliomyelitis
involving the right lower extremity with 1-1/2 inches of shortening on this side. He has a fairly good quadriceps and hamstrings and very good power in the calf muscles, but he has no
anterior tibial or peroneal power at all, nor can I make out any
power in his posterior tibial, this may just be weak. He should
have a stabilization of his right foot, probably a Lambrinudi
operation as recommended by Dr. Goldner, and, at some later
date, an epiphyseal arrest at the left knee. There is no evidence
of scoliosis as yet, but he does have a rather tight iliotibial band

on the right which should be observed further while in the hospital. Dr. Babb.

1-12-50
I would like this boy put on the surgical list for stabilization of his right foot – Lambrinudi operation. At the same time plan to staple distal femoral epiphysis on the left. Dr. Babb.

1-12-50
Scheduled for Lambrinudi operation, stabilization of his right foot and staple distal femoral epiphysis on the left. January 16, 1950 at 10:30 A.M. Dr. Babb.

1-16-50
ANESTHETIC: Pentothal-curare, nitrous oxide
DURATION OF OPERATION Began: 11:25 A.M. Ended 1:45 P.M.
DESCRIPTION OF OPERATION: The foot, ankle and leg were prepared and draped in a sterile manner and a pneumatic tourniquet was applied. A straight horizontal incision was made over the lateral aspect of the right foot. The areolar tissue was removed from the sinus tarsi. With a wide chisel the head of the astragalus was removed together with a wedge from the inferior body of the astragalus. The cartilage was removed from the remainder of the talonavicular joint, from the calcaneocuboid joint and from the talocalcaneal joint. The opposing raw bone surfaces were then fitted together and held with three wire staples. Cancellous bone which had been removed was packed between the opposing bone surfaces. The skin was closed and a long leg plaster cast was applied with the knee in moderate flexion. Immediate postoperative condition was good.
OPERATOR: F.S. Babb, M.D.

1-16-50
Returned from surgery at 2 P.M. Very restless. ... Codeine Sulphate grains 1/2 (h) given at 6:45 P.M. for pain.

1-17-50
Codeine Sulphate grains 1/2 (m) given at 4:30 A.M and 12:15
P.M. and 4:45 P.M. for pain. Codeine Sulphate grains 1/2 (h)
given at 8:45 A.M. Has had considerable pain in right foot and
left knee today.

1-18-50
Codeine Sulphate grains 1/2 and Aspirin grains 10 given at
3:45 A.M. and 2:30 P.M. and 9 P.M. ... S.S. enema given with
very good results.

1-19-50
Aspirin grains 10 given at 12:30 P.M. and 6:45 P.M. with relief.

1-20-50
Aspirin grains 10 given at 2 P.M.

1-21-50
Aspirin grains 10 given at 1 A.M. for discomfort in right foot.

1-26-50
X-ray of the left knee of January 23 shows the distal end of the
femur to be stapled in the usual manner. The staples on the
medial side are a little too low and this knee should be watched
for a knock-knee deformity. Post operative x-rays of the right
foot show the foot following Lambrinudi to be in only a fair position. A little too much of the navicular bone has been removed,
and the foot has been flattened considerably. At the next
change of plaster, an attempt should be made to try to restore
the lateral arch to prevent a rocker bottom foot. Breakfast is to
be withheld next Tuesday when this is to be done. Dr. Babb

1-31-50
Breakfast withheld. Returned from surgery. No complaints of
discomfort following change of cast.

2-1-50
Transferred to Ward 6. Allowed up in wheel chair by order of
Dr. Spray.

2-3-50
Started School.

2-7-50
Patient has had a fever of approximately 103° most of today. ...
Recommended isolation, possible mumps. ... Transferred to
Admitting Unit at 8:15 P.M.

2-9-50
Temperature normal today. Feeling much better.

2-10-50
May be released from isolation.

2-13-50
Transferred to Ward 6.

2-16-50
X-ray on January 31, right foot, shows the position of the
arthrodesis to be unchanged and the three staples in satisfactory position. He has a flexion contracture of the left knee following his stapling operation and is badly in need of quadriceps
exercises. Should attend physio for quadriceps exercises to his
left knee. Will get him a walking cast on the right foot in about
two weeks. Dr. Babb

3-1-50
Up walking on cast with walking iron attached.

3-16-50
The contracture of the left knee does not seem to be improving.
Would recommend that the resident schedule him for an anes-

thetic and see if the knee comes straight. ... If the knee does come straight he is to have a stovepipe plaster applied. The plaster on the right is to be changed at the same time. Dr. Babb.

3-17-50
Patient cancelled for surgery today. Scheduled for Monday, March 20.

3-20-50
No breakfast. Morphine Sulphate grains 1/2 and Atropine Sulphate grains 1/200 given at 11:15 A.M. To surgery at 11:15 A.M.
OPERATION: Manipulation of left knee.
Under relaxation with administration of pentothal and curare, the weight of the leg alone was enough force to straighten our the left knee when the left heel was supported. Accordingly, the leg was maintained with the knee in the straight position and a cylinder cast was applied from the upper thigh to the upper ankle.
Returned at 12:50 awake.

3-22-50
Up and around ...

3-23-50
Seen. Dr. Babb.

3-24-1950
PSYCHOLOGICAL REPORT
COUNTY Ramsey
Handicaps none for testing
Test used Stanford-Binet

Summary
Richard took an immediate interest in the test and appeared to be enthusiastic and alert in his responses. Basal age is nine

years with tests passed through the fourteen year level.
Abstract verbal and concrete-performance ability are developing about evenly. In addition, Richard shows a rather highly
developed social sense on items which require insight into
absurd situations – actions and speech also indicate better than
average social intelligence. His over-all IQ is that of a person
with normal intelligence.

3-30-50
Seen. Dr. Babb.

4-6-50
Seen. Dr. Babb.

4-13-50
To have cast removed from left leg and resume active exercises
for left knee. Remove cast on right leg for next Thursday and
have x-rays of foot out of plaster. Dr. Babb.

4-19-50
Plasters removed.

4-20-50
The right foot is not too good a result. He still has some equinus
and there is a moderate rocker bottom deformity. X-ray shows
what appears to be bony union of his arthrodesis. Is to attend
physiotherapy for active exercises of his left knee and right
foot. To include instruction in walking. Put a felt pad in his
shoes. Dr. Babb.

4-21-50
Up and around in a wheelchair.

5-4-50
He is still having persistent flexor contractions of about 20° in
his left knee. The knee is warmer than the right and becoming

painful. I can only explain this on a basis of traumatic synovitis. I would like him to have another long leg stove pipe plaster applied under ancsthesia with the knee on full extension. X-ray of the left knee on 4-26-50 is not remarkable except for one staple being too far posterior. Dr. Babb.

5-9-50
To surgery at 7:30 A.M.
OPERATION: The patient was anesthetized and it was found that the left knee could be brought into full extension, lacking only two or three degrees. A stovepipe plaster was applied extending from the upper thigh to just above the ankle. Returned at 8 A.M. awake and condition good.

5-18-20
He is to have his right shoe built up 1-1/2 inches in the sole with heel to match and may then be up and walking. Dr. Babb.

5-25-50
He walks pretty well with built up shoe. Would like to try again taking his plaster off the left leg and see if we could keep his knee straight. Save the back half of the plaster and use it as a night splint. Dr. Babb.

6-1-50
His knee now completely extends and flexes to about 135°. I would like him to return to physiotherapy for some more active exercises for his left knee. Dr. Babb.

6-8-50
The left knee is now quite normal. Completely extends. He does not have a very good result in his right foot. He still has a partial drop foot, but it is well healed, no pain. I would ... consider discharge.
Dr. Babb

6-14-50
Complained of headache after the picnic.

6-15-50
X-rays of the right foot taken on June 12th shows what
appears to be a satisfactory stabilization. Clinically, however,
his foot is in a little too much valgus and his foot drop is not
well corrected. He is wearing a built up shoe with a leather
insole on the right which is satisfactory. May be discharged,
home, improved. Dr. Babb.

6-17-50
Discharged to Mother at 1:45 P.M. walking wearing shoes.
Right shoe 1-1/2 inches built up sole and heel to match.

DISCHARGE #3

1-4-51
This patient has a very definite droop foot on the right. He complains of occasional pain in the left knee. Examination shows
no evidence of the staples backing out. The arthrodesis of the
right foot is holding very well, but there is a definite foot drop
and I think a posterior bone block should be considered. Dr.
Hall.

4-17-51
... He will need something further to correct his foot drop and
although he has a trace of power in his peroneals, he has no
other available tendons, right, and I believe a posterior bone
block is his only hope. Is to report when school is out for possible admission.
Dr. Babb.

Chapter 4

ADMISSION #4

7-10-51
Patient comes in now for operative correction of a right foot drop. His interval history is negative. There has been no history of illnesses or injuries.
PREOPERATIVE DIAGNOSIS: A drop foot, right, following a Lambrinudi procedure done in January, 1950.
Admitted to Ward 6
Started school

7-16-51
Transferred to Ward 1. S.S. enema – effectual

7-17-51
Operation began: 11:00 A.M.
DESCRIPTION OF OPERATION: A four-inch vertical incision was made on the posterior aspect of the right leg extending from the calf down to the heel. This incision was made over an old incision done on previous surgery. The incision was extended through scar tissue down to the neurovascular bundle. The posterior tibial nerve and artery were identified and both retracted medially. One tendon was identified lateral to that, which appeared to be the flexor Hallucis longus. No other tendons were identified except for the Achilles tendon, which was retracted laterally. The incision was extended down to the bone, and a site was selected for removal of a square of bone for the bone block. Then the lower part of the incision was extended down through the soft tissues to the bone. The small bleeders were tied off, and the tibiotalar joint was identified. It was also felt that there was a small amount of motion between the astragalus and the calcaneus. It was decided to make vertical groove into the calcaneus to receive the bone block, and this

was performed. Then attention was turned to the tibia about two inches above the epiphyseal line where a 1-1/2 x 1 centimeter square was removed by the use of a handchuck with a small drill point followed by an osteotome and hammer. This piece of bone was then placed in the vertical groove fashioned in the calcaneus, and it was decided to hold it in place by use of a Kirschner wire. After the insertion of the Kirschner wire, the periosteum was sewed back over the tibia and the wound was closed in layers using #00 chromic catgut for the subcutaneous and #00 silk for the skin. Throughout this procedure the foot had been held at exactly 90° on two sandbags. The wound was covered with a sterile dressing, and sterile sheet wadding was then applied over that. A plaster cast was applied from the toes to the vicinity of the tibial tuberosity with the foot held at 90°. After the plaster was applied, the Kirschner wire was cut down to the level of the plaster and a little plaster cup was placed over it so that it would not fall out or be drawn back into the bone by being hit against some object. The patient withstood the procedure well and left the operating room in good condition. F.S. Babb M.D. Operation ended:12:25 P.M. ANESTHETIC: Pentothal-curare, nitrous oxide. Intravenous and inhalation.

7-24-51
Up in a wheelchair

7-31-51
On a fishing trip today

8-2-51
Bumped head against cubical. Small cut on left side of forehead.

8-4-51
Cast on leg loose. To remain in bed.

8-7-51

Operative cast removed, sutures removed. Wound healed well.
Skin-tight plaster applied and covered with aire-lite. X-rays
taken.

8-9-51

Up in wheelchair

8-16-51

Discharged to father at 3:10 P.M.
Discharged, improved, using crutches. Is not to have weightbearing on the right foot. He is to return the first Tuesday in
September for change of cast and application of a short leg
walking cast. Dr. Babb.

DISCHARGE #4

9-4-51

His bone graft is in good position but has not started to be
hypertrophied as yet and may not be united to the os calcis. ...
after this a short leg walking cast can be applied with the ankle
at a right angle for the right foot. Is to return in six weeks for
removal of cast and new X-rays. Dr. Babb.

10-23-51

He should have another short leg right walking cast for his leg
for at least another month and be seen again in five weeks, if
the cast will last that long.

11-27-51

He is four months post-operative. The foot still plantar flexes
about 30° from a right angle, and the X-ray shows no hypertro-
phy of the graft. I see no reason for further immobilization.
There is probably less than 1/4 inch of shortening on the right
so that he will not need any buildup of his right shoe and in fact
he must be watched carefully for removal of staples of the left
knee. Dr. Babb.

3-4-52

Measurements from the anterior superior spine to the medial malleolus revels that the two legs appear to measure equal length today and we must be on the alert to remove the staples from his left knee should this leg get a little short. X-rays of the left knee shows six staples in the distal femoral epiphysis. The right foot still drops and a posterior bone block appears ineffective. This foot drop on the right should probably be corrected even if it means doing another bone block and one might also consider a tenodesis of the anterior tibial tendon right. He should report in a few weeks or else next Tuesday, for admission: Dr. Babb.

ADMISSION #5

3-11-52

Admitted to Hospital 9:00 A.M.

Admitted at noon to ward in wheelchair. Bath and shampoo given.

ORTHOPEDIC PHYSICAL

Patient is a 13 year old well developed, well nourished male child.

Patient walks with a right dropfoot gait.

UPPER EXTREMITIES: There is no residual of poliomyelitis.

LOWER EXTREMITIES: The lower extremities measured from the anterior superior spine to the medial malleolus are equal. The right thigh measures 2-1/4 inches less than the left thigh 5 inches above the patella. The right calf measures 2-1/4 inches less than the left calf 5 inches below the patella. Patient has good muscle power in flexors, extensors, abductors and adductors of the hip. He has good flexors and extensors at the knee. Plantar flexion of the foot is present and of fair quality, although rather markedly weakened when compared with the left. He has no dorsiflexion of the right foot. There is a trace of dorsiflexion of the toes.

3-18-52
Is on the list for surgery for posterior bone block, right foot for
Tuesday, April 1. The graft will have to be taken from the good
tibia, left. Dr. Babb

3-25-52
Is to be scheduled for posterior bone block, right foot for
Tuesday, April 1 at 8:00 A.M. Dr. Babb.

3-31-52
Routine skin preparation. S.S. enema effectual. Nembutal
grains 1 at 9 P.M.

4-1-52
Nembutal grains 1 at 6:30 A.M. Morphine grains 1/8 and
Atropine grains 1/200 at 7: A.M.
To surgery at 7:50 A.M.
DESCRIPTION OF OPERATION: The patient was placed in the
prone position; and under general anesthesia, with the right
side built up on sandbags, the left leg was raised from the table
and bent at the knee so that from the knee to the foot the leg
enjoyed a vertical position. A three-inch incision was made on
the anterior aspect of the left tibia and was continued immediately through the deep fascia to the bone. A Luck saw was used
to cut out a piece of cortical bone 2-1/2 inches in length and 1/2
inch thick in width. The periosteum was then sutured together
and the skin was sutured with #00 silk in a running lock
suture. Following this, dry dressings were placed over the
wound. Sheet wadding was applied over this, and a sterile Ace
bandage was wrapped from below the knee down to the toes of
the left foot.

Then the operator's attention was turned to the right
foot. A three-inch incision was made through the old scar, and
part of the old scar was cut out at the lower end. The incision
was developed so that the Achilles tendon was identified. It
was found that there was much scar tissue on the dorsal

aspect of the tendon, and this was all cleaned away. When the tendon was sectioned, Allis forceps were clamped on the two cut ends and they were retracted out of the field. Below this there was a layer of fat, and the operator went through that down to the bone.

The peroneal tendons were retracted laterally and the other flexor tendons were retracted medially. The former bone block was found. It was weak, and there was a pseudarthrosis in the calcaneal insertion of the block. This was removed, and the hole in the calcaneus was enlarged. With the assistant holding the foot at right angles, the new piece of bone was pounded down into the calcaneus so that it was firmly anchored in the calcaneus and extended very nicely up behind the tibia. The bone was found to be so long that it interfered with the tendons which were to run over it, so about 1/2 inch was cut off and this, too, was pounded into the calcaneus to make the graft much firmer. Small bone fragments were then added; and, following this, the wound was closed in layers with #00 silk used in an interrupted suture for closure of the skin. Dry dressings were then placed over the wound, and the leg was wrapped with sheet wadding. Then the patient was turned over into the supine position. A plaster cast was applied from below the knee to the toes of the right foot. Throughout this whole time an assistant was most careful to hold the foot at a right angle. Patient withstood the procedure well and left the operating room in good condition. The entire procedure was done under tourniquet applied to both thighs.

Returned to ward 10-:30 A.M. Pulse good quality. Large emesis.

4-2-52
Codeine grains 1 at 2 A.M, 7 A.M., 9:40 A.M., 2:45 P.M.(by mouth), 10:00 P.M. for pain.

4-3-52
Codeine grains 1 at 9:45 A.M., 1:15 P.M., for pain
11:00 P.M. no relief from pain. Cast split by Dr Kelley

4-4-52
Temperature still elevated.
Codeine grains 1 at 2:45 A.M., 12:30 P.M., 9:00 P.M. for pain.

4-5-52
S.S. enema effectual
Codeine grains 1 and aspirin grains 10 at 2 P.M.
Cast split all the way by Dr Kelley.
Codeine grains 1 and aspirin grains 10 at 9:15 P.M.
Temperature 102.2°-104.2°

4-6-52
Aspirin grains 10 at 1:30 A.M. and 1:00 P.M. Temperature still
elevated. Codeine grains 1 and Aspirin grains 10 at 7:45 P.M.

4-7-52
There is inflammation in the nasopharynx. This probably
accounts for his temperature elevation.
Aspirin grains 10 at 6:15 A.M. and 1:30 P.M. Petrologar, 1/2
ounce, at 8 P.M. Aspirin grains 10 at 8:30 P.M. for pain in heel.
Codeine grains 1 at 11:30 P.M.

4-8-52
He has been running a post-operative fever between 100° and
102° and complaining of pain in the back of the right heel and
has tender and enlarged inguinal glands in the right groin. This
would seem like sufficient evidence to warrant removal of his
cast and inspection of his wound on the right foot.
Later: His cast was removed, and profusely thick brownish pus
exudated from the upper end of the wound. The upper two
sutures were removed. The wound was spread open and a large
abscess evacuated. A new padded short leg cast was applied
and he is to be kept at bed rest with the leg elevated and
receive Penicillin 100,000 units every three hours and either
Chloremycin or Aureomycin whichever is available. Dr. Babb.
Codeine grains 1 at 10:20 A.M. for pain in heel. To surgery –

cast on right leg changed by Dr Babb.
Penicillin 100,000 units every three hours started at 3 P.M.
Sutures removed from left leg by Dr. Kelley.

4-12-52
Temperature normal.

4-16-52
To surgery. Sutures removed and cast changed, on right leg.

4-22-52
Crysticillin discontinued

14-28-52
Offensive odor from cast on right leg.

4-29-52
Cast on right leg changed. Temperature elevated.
Crysticillin 300,000 U. daily started.

4-30-52
Temperature elevated. Complains of feeling dizzy.

5-6-52
Crysticillin discontinued. Up in chair. Transferred to Ward 6

5-7-52
Up on crutches.

5-13-52
Patient had cast removed with Dr. Babb in attendance. The
area of the wound is healing well with about four small granu-
lating areas remaining. These were cauterized with silver
nitrate and a new skin tight plaster cast applied from below the
knee to the toes over double layer stockinette. Kept in bed until
cast is dry.

5-20-52
Schedule for change of cast for Tuesday, May 27, and possible application of walking cast. No anesthesia. Dr Babb.

5-26-52
Feeling better. Good day.

5-27-52
Is to be scheduled for change of cast next Tuesday, June 3, if it is not done before that time.

6-3-52
Although it is two months post-operative, in view of his wound infection, we will postpone walking in a walking cast for another month. He may be discharged improved on crutches and is to return in one month for removal of cast and x-rays of the right ankle and we will consider application of a short leg walking cast. Is not to bear weight. Dr. Babb.

6-7-52
Discharged, improved. It is two months postoperative, but in view of his wound infection, we will postpone walking in a walking cast for another month. Is to use crutches and is to return in one month for removal of cast and X-ray of the right ankle. We will consider application of a short leg walking cast. Is not to bear weight on the right foot.

DISCHARGE #5

ADMISSION #6

7-1-52
His operative incision is draining again. There is no question but that he will have to be readmitted and the wound, right foot, explored. Remove the silk sutures remaining in the wound. Is to be started on continuous warm moist sterile

dressings to the right heel cord area for 48 hours, then dry dressings. Is to have a hemoglobin, white count, sedimentation rate, and urinalysis. Is to be scheduled for next Tuesday, July 8, for exploration of wound, right foot. Is to be last on list. Dr. Babb.

7-3-52
Suture came out on dressing. Saline packs to foot discontinued after 48 hours. Dry dressing applied.

7-8-52
OPERATION: Exploration of draining sinus, right heel.

7-14-52
OPERATION: Delayed primary closure of wound, right heel.

7-15-52
A good night. Intake 400 c.c. output 350 c.c.

8-20-52
Up in wheelchair. To School.

9-2-52
OPERATION: Excision of scar over Achilles tendon, right. Returned at 2:45 P.M. Awake. Condition good.

9-3-52
No complaints. To school in a wheelchair.

9-9-52
Transferred to Ward 6. Dressings changed, crutches ordered.

9-11-52
Dressings changed. Some serious drainage.

9-15-52
Incision touched up with silver nitrate.

9-16-52

His incision at long last is almost completely healed. He may
start getting up now wearing the shoes he came in with and
start graded weightbearing in physiotherapy. He will require
just a dry protective dressing on his right ankle.
Measurements from the anterior superior spine to the sole of
the heel reveal that there is no gross difference in leg length.
He does not need any shoe build-up now. He does have a little
genu valgus of the left knee. I would like an AP and lateral
x-ray of the left knee for comparison with previous films. May
be up in the ward when ready. Dr. Babb.

9-24-52

X-rays of the left knee reveal a slight increase in the genu valgus. I believe he should have the staples removed from the lateral side of the knee before they are removed from the medial
side and will review the situation in six months with this in
mind. May be discharged, improved. Should be seen again in
one month in OPD. Is to use crutches until we see him again.
Needs transportation to school. Dr. Babb.

9-24-52
Discharged on crutches to parents at 12:15 P.M.

DISCHARGE #6

Chapter 5

ADMISSION #7

1-6-53
PHYSICAL EXAMINATION
The right lower extremity smaller than left, but of equal length.
Scars of previous surgery well healed and non-tender; good
muscle strength. Left leg assumes a genu valgus attitude due to
regrowth on medial side of femoral epiphysis.

Post poliomyelitis involving right leg.
Genu valgus left knee.
DIAGNOSIS: Genu valgus left, residuals of polio lower extremities.

1-6-53
The right foot and ankle are fine except that another little
piece of bone has now come out posteriorly and there is no indications for treatment. His left knee is in more and more valgus
and his left lower extremity is 2 cm. shorter than the right. I
believe the staples should be removed from the distal femoral
epiphysis at the left knee, removed from the lateral side only.
Is to be readmitted and put on the surgery list for Tuesday,
January 13. Dr. Babb.

1-6-53
Admitted at noon. Walked In.

1-13-53
OPERATION: Removal of staples, lateral side of left lower
femoral epiphysis removal of staples and restapling, medial
side of left lower femoral epiphysis.

1-31-53
Crutches discontinued.

2-18-53
Discharged, improved.

DISCHARGE #7

6-4-53
Measurements from the anterior superior spine to the medial
malleolus reveal that the patient has 1 inch of shortening on
the left. Patient still has a draining sinus in the region of the
right heel cord, which is occasionally spitting out a piece of
bone through the draining sinus. Deformity of the left knee

appears to be about the same. Should use the foot powder in his shoes. Can wear ordinary work shoes for every day, high top and they require no special buildup or lift. Patient should return in the fall at which time we should have an AP and Lateral X-ray of the right ankle.

ADMISSION #8

10-6-53
He has had no drainage from the right ankle for two months. Has had no pain. He has quite a marked genu valgus on the left, which measures 20 degrees today. He is acutely tender over the medial femoral condyle of the left knee where the staples appear to be backing out. This is the present problem for which he must be admitted at once. X-rays of the left knee, AP and L and right foot and ankle should be taken. Is to be scheduled for Tuesday, October 13, for removal of the staples and further epiphyseal arrest at the left knee. Dr, Babb.

10-6-53
Admitted walking to Ward 6. Accompanied by mother.

10-13-53
OPERATION: Removal of previously inserted staples, medial epicondyle, left femur, and Phemister operation, medial epicondyle, left femur.

10-13-53
DESCRIPTION OF OPERATION: Excising the previous scar, an incision was made over the medial condyle of the left femur about three inches long in a longitudinal direction. The incision was developed down through the subcutaneous fascia to scar tissue overlying the bone. The previously inserted staples were found and removed. The periosteum over the bone was freed up in this area, and a rectangular piece of bone about one inch long and 3/8 inch wide was raised up in the area of the previously

inserted staples. The epiphyseal line was visualized clearly
going through the region of the previously removed
rectangular piece of bond. The epiphyseal line was curetted out
thoroughly. The rectangular piece of bone was inverted so that
its inferior end was placed superiorly. The fascia was closed
with #000 chromic suture. The skin was closed with #000 silk.
A snug fitting pressure dressing held on by an Ace bandage
wound from the toes to the mid-portion of the femur was
applied. A posterior knee splint was placed over this dressing.
Patient tolerated the procedure well. Operation was performed
under tourniquet and general anesthesia.

10-20-53
Measured for crutches.

10-21-53
To school on crutches.

11-3-53
May start getting up on crutches and in addition to this is to
have non weight bearing quadriceps exercises for the left knee.
Does not need the posterior splint. Dr. Babb.

11-10-53
He has a good quadriceps on the left with complete extension of
his knee. He walks well. May be discharged, improved.
Continue quadriceps exercises for both lower extremities. May
go to school. Needs transportation which his father provides.
He is to be seen in three months. ... Dr. Babb.

11-13-53
Discharged to mother, walking with crutches at 1:00 P.M.

DISCHARGE #8

2-16-54
Right leg measures 1/2 to 3/4 inch longer as measured from
anterior superior iliac spine to internal malleolus. His left
quadriceps are normal as are his hamstrings. Patient has no
complaints. However, he states that occasionally a small piece
of bone will come out through a scar situated posteriorly over
the tendo-Achilles. Should have an x-ray of that. The new x-
rays show a slight overgrowth of bone posteriorly in the ankle
with a possible fragment which seems to be a little denser than
the rest of the bone and may well represent another fragment
of bone which will be discharged. No open sinus is present.
Patient advised to return if any further spicules of bone appear.
Otherwise return in 3 months at which time he should have
another x-ray.

5-11-54
X-RAY READING: X-ray of the right foot and ankle shows the
posterior bone block to be firmly consolidated in a satisfactory
position. Left knee – complete closure of the distal femoral epiphysis with a rather marked genu valgus deformity. This
patient will require a supracondylar osteotomy to correct his
knock knee. Dr. Babb.

6-14-55
He now has a 1/2 inch of shortening on the left side which,
however is partially attributable to a rather marked genu valgus at the left knee which clinically measures 20 degrees. It
was previously noted a supracondylar osteotomy of the left
femur is anticipated. He may be added to the surgical list for
supracondylar osteotomy on the left femur ss soon as there is
room on the surgery schedule. In the meantime I would like
him to have x-rays of both knees, AP and lateral. In the case of
the x-ray of the left knee, this should be on a large 14 x 17 film
with the knee centered. Dr. Babb.

6-14-55
X-ray 14 x17 (rt. Knee, lt. knee)

6-28-55
X-RAY READING: An x-ray of the right knee is normal and the epiphysis appears to be almost closed, X-ray of the left knee reveals the epiphysis to be closed, particularly the distal femoral epiphysis. There is a marked genu valgus present due apparently to overgrowth of the distal femoral epiphysis on the medial side. There is no deformity of the tibia. He can be scheduled for a supracondylar osteotomy of the left femur on Tuesday, July 19. I would anticipate doing the osteotomy from the lateral side and using a block of bone from the adjacent femur to keep the wedge open. Dr. Babb.

Chapter 6

ADMISSION #9

7-12-55
READMITTED
DIAGNOSIS: Residual anterior poliomyelitis, right lower extremity. Dr. Babb.
INTERVAL HISTORY: He is admitted at this time for an osteotomy of the left femur. The interval history reveals the child had mumps in the past year. Had a severe cold with sinusitis approximately three weeks ago. Otherwise his general health has been excellent.

7-19-55
OPERATION: (1) Supracondylar osteotomy, left femur. F. S. Babb. M. D.
Under general anesthetic, with the pneumatic tourniquet in place, the left leg was prepared and draped in the usual fashion. By means of a lateral incision, the fascia lata was exposed. Then, by means of blunt and sharp dissection, the fascia lata

was followed down to the inter-muscular septum. The muscle attachments in this region were then freed exposing the distal end of the femur. Multiple drill holes were then made across the femur in an oblique fashion.

An osteotome was utilized to complete the transection of the bone. With some difficulty the fragments were then levered into position. The difficulty was due to a partial spike remaining on the postero-medial aspect of the distal fragment. The fascia was then closed utilizing one chromic; the skin was closed with interrupted Pyoktanin sutures. (The subcutaneous tissue was closed with #00 plain suture). A pressure dressing was applied and the extremity was immobilized in a spica. However, in the process of the immobilization the fragments were felt to become unlocked. An x-ray taken at this time proved that the distal fragment had slipped posteriorly and proximally. In consequence, a wedge of the spica was removed and an attempt was made to manipulate the fragment into position. However, this proved unsuccessful. In consequence, the plaster was repaired and it was decided to put the patient in traction at a later date to achieve the desired position.

7-28-55
OPERATION: (2) Insertion of Steinman pin, the proximal end of the left tibia.
Under a general anesthetic, the left knee and calf were prepared and draped in the usual fashion. A Steinman pin was then inserted through the proximal third of the tibia. A paraplast dressing was applied and a traction bow fixed. The patient was then placed in balance traction and returned to his room in good condition.

8-4-55
OPERATION: (3) Insertion of Kirschner wire , distal end of left femur.
Under local anesthesia and with x-ray control a Kirschner wire was inserted through the proximal end of the distal fragment of the left femur. It should be noted that a satisfactory inser-

tion of the Kirschner were could not be obtained due to the prior surgery and the position of the distal fragment.

8-9-55
OPERATION: (4) Manipulation of left knee under anesthetic. Under general anesthetic an attempt was made to manipulate the distal fragment from its posterior position. This, however was not successful and, in consequence, the patient was returned to his room in traction.

8-16-55
OPERATION: (5) Open reduction and internal fixation, left femur, for correction of genu valgus. F. S. Babb. M. D.
Under a general anesthetic and with a pneumatic tourniquet in place, the left leg was prepared and draped in the usual manner. The old incision was then opened exposing the fracture site. There was a huge amount of hard callous formation about the fracture ends. The distal fragment was still posterior not reduced.
The fracture area was then cleaned of all callous material and a reduction performed. After ascertaining good reduction a Moe-plate was put in place utilizing two wood screws at this lower and two regular screws in the upper end. The leg was held in the corrected position while fixation was accomplished. The stabilization was fairly good. A small amount of cancellous bone bank bone was then packed in the fracture site, bridging the open wedge on the lateral side. The fascia was then closed in the usual manner.

9-12-55
DISCHARGED, Improved. He will not be able to attend school but I understand his assignments will be sent home to him. He is to return in 6 weeks and be admitted to have cast bivalved and checkup x-rays of the femur to include the knee, taken out of plaster. Dr. Babb.

DISCHARGE #9

9-13-55
The last x-ray shows the knock knee deformity to be well corredted and his knee is now nice and straight, Dr. Babb.

ADMISSION #10

9-19-55
The patient is readmitted at this time because of a broken cast. TREATMENT: Spica cast, dentistry, x-rays.

9-20-55
He had only been home 4 days when his spica cast broke at the osteotomy site. He is to have his cast removed and a new spica cast reapplied and especially reinforced over the osteotomy site.

10-1-55
DISCHARGED, Improved.
To report to the Outpatient Department on Tuesday, November 8, 1955 at 9:00 A.M. for removal of cast and x-rays. Dr. Babb.

DISCHARGE #10

11-8-55
The knee is clinically well healed. ... He should be seen again in about one month to six weeks for further x-rays before unprotected weight bearing is permitted. Discontinue shoe build-up.

4-2-57
Has no complaints. He is now 17 years old. Left leg measures 1/4 inch short compared to the right. His genu valgus on the right is 5°; on the left 10°. By x-ray his preoperative genu valgus on the left measures 16° and now measures 13°. This does

not represent as much improvement on x-ray as it does clinically. However, there is no further treatment indicated at the
present time. See again in two years. Dr. Babb.

3-31-59
Letter to pt.: The x-rays of your knee have been reviewed and
compared with films of two years ago. There is no irritation
around the metal and there seems no indication at present to
remove the plate or screws. If difficulty arises in the future I
would suggest you contact an orthopedist and have the plate
removed. Dr. Babb

About the author

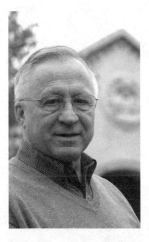

In front of Michael J. Dowling Memorial Hall, formerly part of Gillette and now owned by the Minnesota Humanities Commission, in 2005

Richard Maus underwent 16 operations and spent a total of 938 days at Gillette State Hospital for Crippled Children after contracting polio in 1939 at the age of four months. He flunked out of two colleges before earning bachelor's degrees in math and physics and a master's in math education at St. Cloud State College in St. Cloud, Minnesota. He received his private pilot's license in 1967.

After teaching math, physics, and computer science for 34 years, Maus retired in 2000 to Northfield, Minnesota, where he and his wife, Donna, have built a home without steps. He remains active, swimming regularly at the local senior center, writing, traveling, flying, baking bread, and volunteering in community activities. They have two grown sons, Paul and Steve.

Books. . . .
The Perfect Gift

Three easy ways to get additional copies of *Lucky One:*

1. Visit your local bookstore

2. Send $19.95 (check or money order) for each *Lucky One* book to:
   luckyonebook.com
   204 West 7th Street, Box 8
   Northfield, MN 55057-2419

   FREE shipping (domestic U.S. ground)
   Please make check payable to Anterior Publishing.
   Minnesota residents add 6.5% ($1.30) sales tax for each book ordered.

3. On the Internet go to:
   www.luckyonebook.com

   Huge discounts on orders for multiple books

   FREE shipping (domestic U.S. ground)
   Ordering is secure and simple.